PUBLIC HEALTH IN THE 21ST CENTURY

PHYSICIAN SELF-REFERRALS

SELECT ANALYSES OF TRENDS AND ISSUES

PUBLIC HEALTH IN THE 21ST CENTURY

Additional books in this series can be found on Nova's website
under the Series tab.

Additional e-books in this series can be found on Nova's website
under the e-book tab.

PUBLIC HEALTH IN THE 21ST CENTURY

PHYSICIAN SELF-REFERRALS

SELECT ANALYSES OF TRENDS AND ISSUES

LOUISE HAMILTON
EDITOR

nova publishers
New York

Library of Congress Cataloging-in-Publication Data

ISBN: 978-1-63463-444-1

Published by Nova Science Publishers, Inc. † New York

CONTENTS

PREFACE

Self-referral occurs when a provider refers patients to entities in which the provider or the provider's family members have a financial interest. Rising Medicare expenditures for PT services have long been of concern, and questions have been raised about the role of self-referral in this growth. This book examines trends in the number of and expenditures for self-referred and non-self-referred Medicare PT services and how provision of these services differs among providers on the basis of whether they self-refer. It also discusses similar trends in cancer treatments, anatomic pathology services, and advanced imaging services.

Chapter 1 - Rising Medicare expenditures for PT services have long been of concern, and questions have been raised about the role of self-referral in this growth. Self-referral occurs when a provider refers patients to entities in which the provider or the provider's family members have a financial interest.

GAO was asked to examine self-referral for PT services and Medicare spending for these services. This report examines (1) trends in the number of and expenditures for self-referred and non-self-referred Medicare PT services and (2) how provision of these services differs among providers on the basis of whether they self-refer. GAO analyzed Medicare Part B claims data from 2004 through 2010 and examined three measures of PT referral for each referring provider: number of PT services referred, number of beneficiaries referred, and number of PT services provided per beneficiary. GAO compared PT referrals for self-referring and non-self-referring providers after accounting for referring provider specialty, Medicare beneficiary practice size, and geographic (urban or rural) location. GAO also compared selected characteristics of the beneficiaries referred by self-referring and non-self-referring providers.

The Department of Health and Human Services stated that it had no comments on a draft of this report.

Chapter 2 - Questions have been raised about selfreferral's role in Medicare Part B expenditures' rapid growth. Self-referral occurs when a provider refers patients to entities in which the provider or the provider's family members have a financial interest. Services that can be self-referred under certain circumstances include IMRT, a common and costly treatment for prostate cancer. GAO was asked to examine Medicare self-referral trends among radiation oncology services. This report examines (1) trends in the number of and expenditures for prostate cancer-related IMRT services provided by self-referring and non-selfreferring provider groups from 2006 through 2010 and (2) how the percentage of prostate cancer patients referred for IMRT may differ on the basis of whether providers self-refer.

GAO analyzed Medicare Part B claims and developed a claims-based methodology to identify self-referring groups and providers. GAO also interviewed officials from the Centers for Medicare & Medicaid Services (CMS), which administers Medicare, and other stakeholders.

Chapter 3 - Questions have been raised about selfreferral's role in Medicare Part B expenditures' rapid growth. Self-referral occurs when providers refer patients to entities in which they or their family members have a financial interest. Services that can be self-referred under certain circumstances include anatomic pathology—the preparation and examination of tissue samples to diagnose disease. GAO was asked to examine the prevalence of anatomic pathology self-referral and its effect on Medicare spending. This report examines (1) trends in the number of and expenditures for self-referred and non-self-referred anatomic pathology services, (2) how provision of these services may differ on the basis of whether providers self-refer, and (3) implications of self-referral for Medicare spending. GAO analyzed Medicare Part B claims data from 2004 through 2010 and interviewed officials from the Centers for Medicare & Medicaid Services (CMS) and other stakeholders. GAO developed a claims-based approach to identify self-referred services because Medicare claims lack such an indicator.

Chapter 4 - Medicare Part B expenditures—which include payment for advanced imaging services—are expected to continue growing at an unsustainable rate. Questions have been raised about selfreferral's role in this growth. Self-referral occurs when a provider refers patients to entities in which the provider or the provider's family members have a financial interest. GAO was asked to examine the prevalence of advanced imaging self-referral and its effect on Medicare spending. This report examines (1) trends in the number of and expenditures for self-referred and nonself-referred advanced imaging services, (2) how provision of these services differs among providers on the basis of whether they self-refer, and (3) implications of self-referral for Medicare spending. GAO analyzed Medicare Part B claims data from 2004 through 2010 and interviewed officials from the Centers for Medicare & Medicaid Services (CMS) and other stakeholders. Because Medicare claims lack an indicator identifying self-referred services, GAO developed a claims-based methodology to identify self-referred services and expenditures and to characterize providers as self-referring or not.

In: Physician Self-Referrals
Editor: Louise Hamilton

ISBN: 978-1-63463-444-1

Chapter 1

MEDICARE PHYSICAL THERAPY: SELF-REFERRING PROVIDERS GENERALLY REFERRED MORE BENEFICIARIES BUT FEWER SERVICES PER BENEFICIARY*

United States Government Accountability Office

WHY GAO DID THIS STUDY

Rising Medicare expenditures for PT services have long been of concern, and questions have been raised about the role of self-referral in this growth. Self-referral occurs when a provider refers patients to entities in which the provider or the provider's family members have a financial interest.

GAO was asked to examine self-referral for PT services and Medicare spending for these services. This report examines (1) trends in the number of and expenditures for self-referred and non-self-referred Medicare PT services and (2) how provision of these services differs among providers on the basis of whether they self-refer. GAO analyzed Medicare Part B claims data from 2004 through 2010 and examined three measures of PT referral for each referring provider: number of PT services referred, number of beneficiaries referred, and number of PT services provided per beneficiary. GAO compared PT referrals for self-referring and non-self-referring providers after accounting for referring provider specialty, Medicare beneficiary practice size, and geographic (urban or rural) location. GAO also compared selected characteristics of the beneficiaries referred by self-referring and non-self-referring providers.

The Department of Health and Human Services stated that it had no comments on a draft of this report.

* This is an edited, reformatted and augmented version of a United States Government Accountability Office publication, No. GAO-14-270, dated April 2014.

WHAT GAO FOUND

From 2004 to 2010, non-self-referred physical therapy (PT) services increased at a faster rate than self-referred PT services. During this period, the number of self-referred PT services per 1,000 Medicare fee-for-service beneficiaries was generally flat, while non-self-referred PT services grew by about 41 percent. Similarly, the growth rate in expenditures associated with non-self-referred PT services was also higher than for self-referred services.

The relationship between provider self-referral status and PT referral patterns was mixed and varied on the basis of referring provider specialty, Medicare beneficiary practice size, and geography. GAO examined three measures of PT referral for each referring provider for the three provider specialties that referred nearly 75 percent of PT services in 2010—family practice, internal medicine, and orthopedic surgery.

- The overall relationship between provider referral status and the first measure of PT referrals—the average number of PT services referred per provider—was mixed. GAO found that self-referring family practice and internal medicine providers in urban areas, on average, generally referred more PT services than their non-self-referring counterparts. In contrast, self-referring orthopedic surgeons, on average, generally referred fewer PT services than non-self-referring orthopedic surgeons.
- Self-referring providers in all three specialties that GAO examined generally referred more beneficiaries for PT services, on average, but for fewer PT services per beneficiary compared with non-self-referring providers. For these two measures of PT referrals, differences between self-referring and non-self-referring providers generally persisted after accounting for referring providers' specialty, Medicare beneficiary practice size, and geographic location, although the magnitude of these differences varied on the basis of these factors. For example, the average number of beneficiaries referred by self-referring family practice providers in urban areas was approximately 43 to 87 percent higher than for their non-self-referring counterparts, depending on Medicare practice size. In contrast, beneficiaries referred by self-referring family practice providers in urban areas received 12 to 28 percent fewer PT services, on average, depending on practice size, compared with their nonself-referring counterparts.
- GAO also found that in the year a provider began to self-refer, PT service referrals increased at a higher rate relative to non-self-referring providers of the same specialty. For example, family practice providers that began self-referring in 2009 increased PT referrals 33 percent between 2008 and 2010. In contrast, non-self-referring family practice providers increased their PT service referrals 14 percent during this same period.

ABBREVIATIONS

AAFP	American Academy of Family Physicians
AAOS	American Academy of Orthopaedic Surgeons
ACP	American College of Physicians

APTA	American Physical Therapy Association
BBA	Balanced Budget Act of 1997
CCS	Clinical Classification Software
CMS	Centers for Medicare & Medicaid Services
FFS	fee-for-service
HCPCS	Healthcare Common Procedure Coding System
ICD-9-CM	International Classification of Diseases, Ninth Revision, Clinical Modification
NPI	national provider identifier
PT	physical therapy
TIN	Taxpayer Identification Number

* * *

April 30, 2014

The Honorable Charles E. Grassley
Ranking Member
Committee on the Judiciary
United States Senate

The Honorable Henry A. Waxman
Ranking Member
Committee on Energy and Commerce
House of Representatives

The Honorable Sander Levin
Ranking Member
Committee on Ways and Means
House of Representatives

Rising Medicare spending for outpatient therapy services, including physical therapy (PT), has long been an issue. Between 2006 and 2009, Medicare expenditures for outpatient PT increased by approximately 28 percent, while the national economy grew about 4 percent. In 2011, Medicare paid about $4.1 billion for outpatient PT services provided to about 4.3 million Medicare beneficiaries. PT services, such as therapeutic exercises, are designed to improve mobility, strength, and physical functioning, and to limit the extent of disability resulting from injury or disease. An aging U.S. population that remains active later than previous generations may have contributed to an increase in demand for such services. However, there is concern that not all PT services may be medically necessary, and selected legislation has focused on reforming how the Centers for Medicare & Medicaid Services (CMS)—the agency that administers the Medicare program—pays for and manages the outpatient therapy benefit. For example, under the Balanced Budget Act of 1997 (BBA), CMS was required to apply per beneficiary financial limits, known as therapy caps, to help control spending growth and discourage medically unnecessary use of outpatient therapy services, including PT.[1] More recently, the Middle Class Tax Relief and Job Creation Act of

2012 required CMS to gather information on patient function during the course of therapy to better understand patient condition and outcomes for outpatient therapy claims, including PT, beginning January 1, 2013.[2]

Some policymakers also have expressed concern that some of the growth in PT may be the result of provider self-referral, which occurs when providers refer their patients for services delivered by entities— such as their own solo or group practice—in which they or a member of their family have a financial relationship.[3] While federal law generally prohibits self-referral under Medicare, there are exceptions for certain services and arrangements, including PT.[4] Opponents of self-referral for PT suggest that financial incentives may lead providers to initiate PT services more frequently than is necessary, leading to overutilization and increased Medicare spending. Proponents of PT self-referral suggest that such arrangements allow providers to improve coordination of care and provide patients with convenient access to PT services. Some proponents also have argued that physical therapists practicing independently can have a financial incentive to recommend additional PT visits and perform more PT procedures per visit than may be medically necessary.

We have recently reported on self-referral for advanced imaging, anatomic pathology, and intensity modulated radiation therapy.[5] We generally found that providers who self-refer tended to use more of these health care services, in some cases resulting in additional Medicare spending. You also asked us to examine provider self-referral for PT services and Medicare spending for these services. In this report, we provide information on (1) trends in the number of and expenditures for self-referred and non-self-referred Medicare PT services from 2004 through 2010 and (2) how provision of these services differs among providers on the basis of whether they self-refer.

To identify trends in the utilization of and expenditures for self-referred and non-self-referred PT services, we analyzed 100 percent of Medicare fee-for-service (FFS) claims from the Medicare Part B Carrier File from 2004 through 2010 for PT services provided in professional offices. 6 Because there is no "indicator" or "flag" on Medicare claims to identify whether PT services are self-referred or non-self-referred, we developed a claims-based methodology for identifying self-referred services. We classified services as self-referred if the provider shown in the referring provider field for PT services and the provider that performed the PT service had a financial relationship with the same entity.[7] We classified services as non-self-referred if the provider shown in the referring provider field for PT services had no financial relationship with the provider who performed the PT service.[8] After we classified PT services as self-referred or non-self-referred, we used the claims to identify trends in the number of self-referred and non-self-referred PT services and expenditures for PT services performed from 2004 through 2010.[9] (See app. I for more details on our scope and methodology.)

To determine the extent to which the referral of PT services differed for providers who self-referred when compared with other providers, we classified providers into subgroups based on characteristics that may be associated with the amount of PT referrals. We then performed two analyses using 100 percent of Medicare Part B claims for PT services provided in both professional offices and facility settings. For the first analysis, we compared PT referrals during 2010 by providers who self-referred at least one beneficiary for PT services ("self-referring" providers) with providers who referred all beneficiaries for PT services to provider(s) with whom they had no financial relationship ("non-self-referring" providers). [10] Because the amount, frequency, and duration of PT services may vary for each beneficiary, we examined three PT referral measures for each referring provider: total number of PT services referred, total number of beneficiaries referred, and average number of PT services received by each beneficiary referred. Differences in these measures of PT referrals between providers may reflect differences due to self-referral status, provider characteristics, or beneficiary characteristics. To account for provider characteristics that may be associated with the amount of PT referrals, we categorized self-referring and non-self-referring providers into subgroups of similar specialties, geographic areas (urban/rural location), and beneficiary practice size (i.e., the number of Medicare FFS beneficiaries treated in a professional office for any medical condition), and examined our three PT referral measures for self-referring and nonself-referring providers of each subgroup.[11] We examined PT referral measures for providers in three specialties that we found referred nearly 75 percent of PT services in 2010—family practice, internal medicine, and orthopedic surgery.[12] To account for differences in beneficiary characteristics, we compared selected characteristics of the beneficiaries referred by self-referring and non-self-referring providers, such as beneficiary age and disability status.

For our second analysis, we analyzed the extent to which the total number of PT services referred changed the year after providers began to self-refer. Specifically, we identified a group of providers that began to self-refer PT services in 2009. We then calculated the difference in the percentage change in the number of PT services referred by two groups of providers—"switchers" and non-self-referring providers. Switchers were non-self-referring during 2008 and self-referring during 2009 and 2010. Switchers may have begun to self-refer in 2009 by hiring PT provider(s) or joining a group practice that self-referred. Non-self-referring providers were providers who were non-self-referring throughout 2008, 2009, and 2010.

Our study has some limitations. First, we may not have identified all self-referred PT services because CMS uses the referring provider identifier on PT claims to identify the provider who certified the beneficiary's plan of care, and in some cases the referring provider may be different from the certifying provider. In addition, Medicare claims data do not capture all financial relationships between performing and referring providers. Second, we may have understated the occurrence of certain self-referral arrangements, such as referring physician ownership of hospitals, by assuming that all PT services referred to facilities were non-self-referred. Third, our analysis that compares PT diagnostic categories for beneficiaries referred by self-referring and non-self-referring providers is based on data that CMS does not use to determine payment for PT services. Consequently, providers do not have a financial incentive to accurately report diagnostic data for PT services on Medicare claims. Finally, it is outside the scope of this report to examine the medical necessity, clinical appropriateness, or effectiveness of PT services beneficiaries received.

We assessed the reliability of the CMS data we used by interviewing officials responsible for overseeing these data sources, reviewing relevant documentation, comparing means and frequencies of selected variables with published data, and examining the data for obvious errors. We determined that the data were sufficiently reliable for the purposes of this report.

We conducted this performance audit from February 2012 through April 2014 in accordance with generally accepted government auditing standards. Those standards require that we plan and perform the audit to obtain sufficient, appropriate evidence to provide a reasonable basis for our findings and conclusions based on our audit objectives. We believe that the evidence obtained provides a reasonable basis for our findings and conclusions based on our audit objectives.

BACKGROUND

PT treatment consists of a planned program to relieve symptoms, improve function, and prevent further disability for individuals disabled by chronic or acute disease or injury. Health conditions that require physical rehabilitation, such as low back pain, bursitis, stroke, Parkinson's disease, or arthritis, may benefit from PT services. Beneficiaries are eligible to receive outpatient PT under Medicare Part B, which covers diagnosis and treatment of impairments, functional limitations, disabilities, or changes in physical function and health status. Medicare-covered outpatient PT services are provided in institutional settings such as hospital outpatient departments and skilled nursing facilities, as well as noninstitutional settings such as physicians' offices and PT clinics.

To be covered by Medicare, outpatient PT services must be medically necessary, furnished while the beneficiary is or was under the care of a physician, and provided under a written plan of care established by an appropriate medical professional, such as a physician or physical therapist. The plan of care is required to contain, among other information, the amount, duration, and frequency of PT services.[13] The plan of care must be certified by a physician or nonphysician practitioner within 30 days of the initial therapy treatment, and must be recertified at least every 90 days after the initial treatment.[14] Medicare does not require that a beneficiary obtain a physician referral to initiate PT services.[15] However, if a physician referral for PT services is documented in the medical record, it provides evidence that the patient was under the care of a physician.

PT services are billed using Healthcare Common Procedure Coding System (HCPCS) codes; examples of HCPCS codes for PT services include therapeutic exercises and massage therapy. Each Medicare claim for PT can include one or more HCPCS codes, as well as one or more 15-minute "units" for each timed code.[16]

SELF-REFERRED PT SERVICES AND EXPENDITURES FROM 2004 THROUGH 2010 WERE GENERALLY FLAT, WHILE NON-SELF-REFERRED PT SERVICES AND EXPENDITURES INCREASED

The total number of PT services provided to Medicare beneficiaries increased nearly 30 percent from 2004 through 2010. Over this period, the number of self-referred PT services was generally flat, while the number of non-self-referred PT services increased. In addition, expenditures increased over this time period for both self-referred and non-self-referred PT services, but this increase was larger for services that were not self-referred.[17]

Self-Referred PT Services Were Generally Flat; NonSelf-Referred Services Increased About 40 Percent

The total number of PT services provided to Medicare beneficiaries increased nearly 30 percent from 2004 through 2010, despite a small decrease in the total number of FFS beneficiaries over this same period.[18] From 2004 to 2010, the number of services per 1,000 FFS beneficiaries that we identified as self-referred was generally flat—about 320 services in both 2004 and 2010 (see figure 1).[19] In contrast, the number of non-selfreferred PT services per 1,000 FFS beneficiaries grew by about 41 percent, from about 903 in 2004 to about 1,275 services in 2010. Because of the rapid growth in non-self-referred PT services, the proportion of PT services that were self-referred decreased from about 24 percent in 2004 to about 18 percent in 2010.

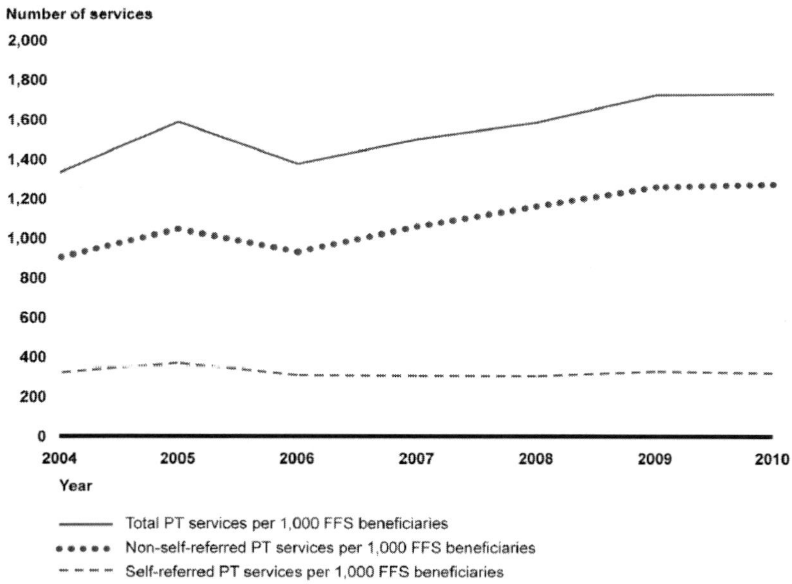

Source: GAO analysis of CMS data.

Note: We analyzed 100 percent of Medicare Part B claims data and counted physical therapy (PT) services based on the number of PT Healthcare Common Procedure Coding System (HCPCS) services on each claim that Medicare covered in a physician office or PT clinic. Total PT services per 1,000 fee-for-service (FFS) beneficiaries include PT services that we could not classify as self-referred or non-self-referred because a referring provider identifier was not included on the Medicare claim. From 2004 to 2010, approximately 8.9 percent of Medicare claims for PT services provided in a physician office or PT clinic did not include a referring provider identifier.

Figure 1. Trends in Number of Self-Referred and Non-Self-Referred Physical Therapy Services per 1,000 Medicare Fee-for-Service Beneficiaries, 2004-2010.

The overall increase in PT services is likely due, in part, to an increase in the proportion of Medicare beneficiaries receiving these services. In 2004, approximately 4 percent of all Medicare FFS beneficiaries received PT services; this increased to approximately 6 percent in 2010. However, from 2004 through 2010, the number of beneficiaries that received self-referred PT services increased only 12 percent, while the number of beneficiaries that received non-self-referred PT services increased nearly 44 percent. In addition, the number of both self-referred and non-self-referred PT services temporarily declined in 2006, likely due to the reinstatement of the therapy payment cap on PT services.[20]

Expenditures for Self-Referred PT Services Increased About 10 Percent; Expenditures for Non-Self-Referred Services Increased Nearly 60 Percent

Expenditures for both self-referred and non-self-referred PT services grew from 2004 to 2010, but the increase was smaller for self-referred services (see figure 2). Specifically, expenditures for self-referred services increased from \$389 million to \$428 million, an increase of about 10 percent. In contrast, expenditures for non-self-referred services increased from \$1.2 billion in 2004 to \$1.9 billion in 2010, an increase of about 57 percent. The larger increase in non-self-referred expenditures from 2004 to 2010 reflects the disproportionate increase in the number of beneficiaries receiving non-self-referred PT services over this period as well as more rapid growth in the number of 15-minute units billed for nonself-referred PT services.[21]

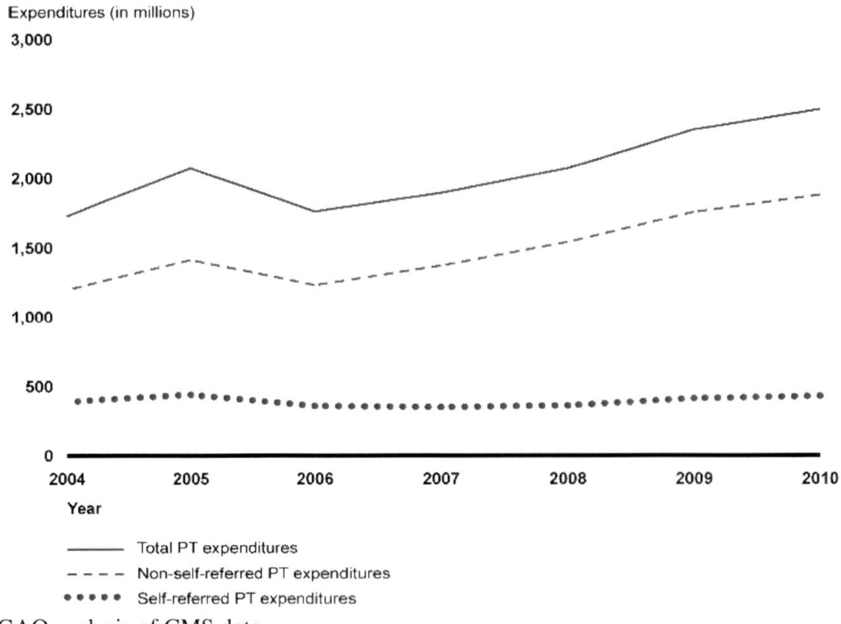

Source: GAO analysis of CMS data.

Note: Medicare expenditures are in nominal dollars. We analyzed 100 percent of Medicare Part B claims data and included all expenditures for physical therapy (PT) Healthcare Common Procedure Coding System (HCPCS) services on each claim that Medicare covered in a physician office or PT clinic. Total PT expenditures include PT services that we could not classify as self-referred or non-self-referred because a referring provider identifier was not included on the Medicare claim. From 2004 to 2010, approximately 8.6 percent of Medicare claims for PT expenditures in a physician office or PT clinic did not include a referring provider identifier.

Figure 2. Trends in Self-Referred and Non-Self-Referred Medicare Physical Therapy Expenditures, 2004-2010.

PT REFERRAL PATTERNS DIFFERED ON THE BASIS OF WHETHER THE PROVIDERS SELF-REFERRED

The overall relationship between provider referral status and the average number of PT services referred per provider was mixed and varied on the basis of referring provider specialty, Medicare beneficiary practice size, and geography. For example, self-referring family practice and internal medicine providers in urban areas, on average, generally referred more PT services in 2010 than their non-self-referring counterparts. Self-referring orthopedic surgeons, on average, generally referred fewer PT services than non-self-referring orthopedic surgeons. In addition, self-referring providers generally referred more beneficiaries for PT services, on average, than non-self-referring providers after accounting for differences in provider specialty, Medicare beneficiary practice size, and geography.[22] However, self-referring providers, on average, referred fewer PT services per beneficiary than non-self-referring providers. Providers' referrals for PT services increased the year after they began to self-refer at a greater rate than non-self-referring providers.

Table 1. Average Number of Medicare Physical Therapy Services Referred in Urban Areas, by Provider Referral Status, Selected Specialty, and Beneficiary Practice Size in 2010

Provider specialty and Medicare beneficiary practice size[a]	Urban self-referring providers	Urban non-self-referring providers	Relative rate of self-referring providers[b]
Family practice			
0 to 50	150.2	119.5	1.26
51 to 100	185.9	129.1	1.44
101 to 250	385.4	276.0	1.40
251 to 500	848.6	625.8	1.36
501+	1,756.3	1,639.2	1.07
Internal medicine			
0 to 50	150.8	175.5	0.86
51 to 100	361.4	143.2	2.52
101 to 250	465.9	309.1	1.51
251 to 500	799.4	679.5	1.18
501+	1,811.4	1,567.5	1.16
Orthopedic surgery			
0 to 50	195.7	243.9	0.80
51 to 100	431.9	442.0	0.98
101 to 250	1,001.4	984.7	1.02
251 to 500	1,892.1	2,034.4	0.93
501+	3,960.3	4,124.8	0.96

Source: GAO analysis of CMS data.

Notes: We analyzed 100 percent of Medicare Part B claims data and counted physical therapy (PT) services based on the number of PT Healthcare Common Procedure Coding System (HCPCS) services on each claim that Medicare covered in a physician office, PT clinic, outpatient hospital department, skilled nursing facility, comprehensive outpatient rehabilitation facility, rehabilitation agency, or home health agency.

We considered providers to be self-referring if they self-referred at least one PT service during 2010 and non-self-referring if they referred at least one PT service to a professional office during 2010 and none of their referrals were self-referred. To identify providers as practicing in urban areas, we used urban-rural commuting area codes, which are a Census-tractbased classification scheme. In 2010, there were 4,869 self-referring providers in family practice, 4,367 in internal medicine, and 6,458 in orthopedic surgery in urban areas. There were 35,977 nonself-referring providers in family practice, 39,981 in internal medicine, and 11,463 in orthopedic surgery in urban areas.

[a]The Medicare beneficiary practice size for each provider refers to the number of unique Medicare fee-for-service (FFS) beneficiaries that received at least one service in a professional office from that provider during 2010 for any medical condition that was covered by Medicare. Some referring providers had a beneficiary practice size of zero because they treated all their Medicare FFS beneficiaries in a setting other than a professional office (such as a hospital outpatient department).

[b]The relative rate of self-referring providers refers to the factor by which the average number of services referred by self-referring providers is different from the average number of services referred by non-self-referring providers. For example, if the relative rate of self-referring providers is equal to 2, it would mean that, on average, self-referring providers referred 2 times as many PT services as did non-self-referring providers.

Table 2. Average Number of Medicare Physical Therapy Services Referred in Rural Areas, by Provider Referral Status, Selected Specialty, and Beneficiary Practice Size in 2010

Provider specialty and Medicare beneficiary practice size[a]	Rural self-referring providers	Rural non-self-referring providers	Relative rate of self-referring providers[b]
Family practice			
0 to 50	226.5	245.8	0.92
51 to 100	222.9	321.5	0.69
101 to 250	311.0	393.4	0.79
251 to 500	682.3	718.7	0.95
501+	1,969.3	1,442.9	1.36
Internal medicine			
0 to 50	211.1	320.0	0.66
51 to 100	415.2	372.2	1.12
101 to 250	405.1	398.4	1.02
251 to 500	567.4	645.6	0.88
501+	1,332.3	1,440.2	0.93
Orthopedic surgery			
0 to 50	169.8	227.7	0.75
51 to 100	213.7	320.7	0.67
101 to 250	667.4	841.5	0.79
251 to 500	1,654.4	1,559.2	1.06
501+	3,069.2	3,222.1	0.95

Source: GAO analysis of CMS data.

Notes: We analyzed 100 percent of Medicare Part B claims data and counted physical therapy (PT) services based on the number of PT Healthcare Common Procedure Coding System (HCPCS) services on each claim that Medicare covered in a physician office, PT clinic, outpatient hospital department, skilled nursing facility, comprehensive outpatient rehabilitation facility, rehabilitation agency, or home health agency.

We considered providers as self-referring if they self-referred at least one PT service during 2010 and non-self-referring if they referred at least one PT service to a professional office during 2010 and none of their referrals were self-referred. To identify providers as practicing in rural areas, we used urban-rural commuting area codes, which are a Census-tract-based classification scheme. In 2010, there were 964 self-referring providers in family practice, 452 in internal medicine, and 596 in orthopedic surgery in rural areas. There were 11,492 non-self-referring providers in family practice, 5,584 in internal medicine, and 2,327 in orthopedic surgery in rural areas.

[a]The Medicare beneficiary practice size for each provider refers to the number of unique Medicare fee-for-service (FFS) beneficiaries that received at least one service in a professional office from that provider during 2010 for any medical condition that was covered by Medicare. Some referring providers had a beneficiary practice size of zero because they treated all their Medicare FFS beneficiaries in a setting other than a professional office (such as a hospital outpatient department).

[b]The relative rate of self-referring providers refers to the factor by which the average number of services referred by self-referring providers is different from the average number of services referred by non-self-referring providers. For example, if the relative rate of self-referring providers is equal to 2, it would mean that, on average, self-referring providers referred 2 times as many PT services as did non-self-referring providers.

Overall Relationship between Provider Referral Status and Average Number of PT Services Referred Was Mixed

In 2010, the relationship between provider referral status and number of PT services referred across all beneficiaries differed on the basis of geography, provider specialty, and Medicare beneficiary practice size. In urban areas, self-referring providers generally referred more PT services, on average, than non-self-referring providers, with some exceptions (see table 1). For example, self-referring family practice providers in urban areas referred more services, on average, than non-self-referring family practice providers in every beneficiary practice size category. In contrast, self-referring orthopedic surgeons in urban areas referred fewer PT services, on average, in every beneficiary practice size category except the middle category (101 to 250 beneficiaries).

In rural areas, self-referring providers in the three specialties generally referred fewer PT services, on average, than non-self-referring providers, with some exceptions, as shown in table 2.[23] For example, self-referring family practice providers with a beneficiary practice size greater than 500, and orthopedic surgeons in rural areas with a beneficiary practice size of 251 through 500 beneficiaries referred more PT services, on average.

In 2010, Self-Referring Providers Generally Referred More Beneficiaries, on Average, but Referred Fewer PT Services per Beneficiary

Self-referring providers generally referred more beneficiaries for PT services during 2010, on average, but referred fewer PT services per beneficiary compared with non-self-referring providers. Specifically, in urban areas, self-referring providers in family practice, internal medicine, and orthopedic surgery referred more beneficiaries for PT services on average, than their non-self-referring counterparts in every Medicare beneficiary practice size category.[24] However, the magnitude of the differences between the two groups varied by specialty and practice size. For example, the average number of beneficiaries referred by self-referring orthopedic surgeons was 13 to 29 percent higher than for their non-self-referring counterparts, depending on the beneficiary practice size category, while the average number of beneficiaries referred by self-referring family practice providers was approximately 43 to 87 percent higher than for their non-self-referring counterparts, depending on the beneficiary practice size category (see table 3).[25]

Table 3. Average Number of Medicare Beneficiary Referrals for Physical Therapy Services in Urban Areas, by Provider Referral Status, Selected Specialty, and Beneficiary Practice Size in 2010

Provider specialty and Medicare beneficiary practice size[a]	Urban self-referring providers	Urban non-self-referring providers	Relative rate of self-referring providers[b]
Family practice			
0 to 50	5.6	4.0	1.43
51 to 100	8.9	4.8	1.87
101 to 250	15.0	8.8	1.71
251 to 500	26.6	16.3	1.63
501+	48.2	32.3	1.49
Internal medicine			
0 to 50	6.7	4.9	1.35
51 to 100	11.5	4.8	2.40
101 to 250	16.9	9.2	1.83
251 to 500	27.2	17.8	1.53
501+	48.8	33.8	1.44
Orthopedic surgery			
0 to 50	8.4	7.4	1.13
51 to 100	18.4	14.4	1.28
101 to 250	39.6	30.8	1.29
251 to 500	72.2	61.5	1.17
501+	140.5	118.7	1.18

Source: GAO analysis of CMS data.

Notes: We analyzed 100 percent of Medicare Part B claims data and counted physical therapy (PT) services based on the number of PT Healthcare Common Procedure Coding System (HCPCS) services on each claim that Medicare covered in a physician office, PT clinic, outpatient hospital department, skilled nursing facility, comprehensive outpatient rehabilitation facility, rehabilitation agency, or home health agency. For this analysis, we considered providers as self-referring if they self-referred at least one PT service during 2010, and as non-self-referring if they referred at least one PT service to a professional office during 2010 and none of their referrals were self-referred. To identify providers as practicing in urban areas, we used urban-rural commuting area codes, which are a Census-tract-based classification scheme. In 2010, there were 4,869 self-referring providers in family practice, 4,367 in internal medicine, and 6,458 in orthopedic surgery in urban areas. There were 35,977 non-self-referring providers in family practice, 39,981 in internal medicine, and 11,463 in orthopedic surgery in urban areas.

[a]The Medicare beneficiary practice size for each provider refers to the number of unique Medicare fee-for-service (FFS) beneficiaries that received at least one service in a professional office from that provider during 2010 for any medical condition that was covered by Medicare. Some referring providers had a beneficiary practice size of zero because they treated all their Medicare FFS beneficiaries in a setting other than a professional office (such as a hospital outpatient department).

[b]The relative rate of self-referring providers refers to the factor by which the average number of services referred by self-referring providers is different from the average number of services referred by non-self-referring providers. For example, if the relative rate of self-referring providers is equal to 2, it would mean that, on average, self-referring providers referred 2 times as many PT services as did non-self-referring providers.

In general, self-referring providers in rural areas also tended to refer more beneficiaries for PT services across provider specialties and practice size categories. In rural areas, self-referring providers in family practice in our smallest beneficiary practice size category and orthopedic surgery with a practice size of 51 to 100 beneficiaries referred fewer beneficiaries for PT services, on average, than their non-self-referring counterparts. However, in all other instances, self-referring providers in rural areas referred more beneficiaries for PT services, on average, than their non-self-referring counterparts. For example, self-referring internal medicine providers in rural areas referred about 25 to 94 percent more beneficiaries than their non-self-referring counterparts, depending on the beneficiary practice size category (see table 4).

Table 4. Average Number of Medicare Beneficiary Referrals for Physical Therapy Services in Rural Areas, by Provider Referral Status, Selected Specialty, and Beneficiary Practice Size in 2010

Provider specialty and Medicare beneficiary practice size[a]	Rural self-referring providers	Rural non-self-referring providers	Relative rate of self-referring providers[b]
Family practice			
0 to 50	7.0	7.1	0.99
51 to 100	12.2	8.6	1.42
101 to 250	15.1	11.4	1.33
251 to 500	24.3	18.1	1.35
501+	49.8	30.6	1.63
Internal medicine			
0 to 50	11.2	7.4	1.51
51 to 100	18.8	9.7	1.94
101 to 250	14.6	11.7	1.25
251 to 500	23.4	17.8	1.31
501+	42.8	32.8	1.30
Orthopedic surgery			
0 to 50	9.8	8.4	1.16
51 to 100	11.5	12.0	0.96
101 to 250	34.0	30.0	1.13
251 to 500	71.1	54.5	1.30
501+	126.6	102.7	1.23

Source: GAO analysis of CMS data.

Notes: We analyzed 100 percent of Medicare Part B claims data and counted physical therapy (PT) services based on the number of PT Healthcare Common Procedure Coding System (HCPCS) services on each claim that Medicare covered in a physician office, PT clinic, outpatient hospital department, skilled nursing facility, comprehensive outpatient rehabilitation facility, rehabilitation agency, or home health agency. For this analysis, we considered providers as self-referring if they self-referred at least one PT service during 2010 and as non-self-referring if they referred at least one PT service to a professional office during 2010 and none of their referrals were self-referred. To identify providers as practicing in rural areas, we used urban-rural commuting area codes, which are a Census-tract-based classification scheme. In 2010, there were 964 self-referring providers in family practice, 452 in internal medicine, and 596 in orthopedic surgery in rural areas. There were 11,492 non-self-referring providers in family practice, 5,584 in internal medicine, and 2,327 in orthopedic surgery in rural areas.

[a]The Medicare beneficiary practice size for each provider refers to the number of unique beneficiaries that received at least one service in a professional office from that provider during 2010 for any medical condition that was covered by Medicare. Some referring providers had a beneficiary practice size of zero because they treated all their Medicare fee-for-service (FFS) beneficiaries in a setting other than a professional office (such as a hospital outpatient department).

[b]The relative rate of self-referring providers refers to the factor by which the average number of services referred by self-referring providers is different from the average number of services referred by non-self-referring providers. For example, if the relative rate of self-referring providers is equal to 2, it would mean that, on average, self-referring providers referred 2 times as many PT services as did non-self-referring providers.

Table 5. Average Number of Physical Therapy Services Received per Medicare Beneficiary in Urban Areas, by Provider Referral Status, Selected Specialty, and Beneficiary Practice Size in 2010

Provider specialty and Medicare beneficiary practice size[a]	Urban self-referring providers	Urban non-self-referring providers	Relative rate of self-referring providers[b]
Family practice			
0 to 50	26.7	30.3	0.88
51 to 100	20.8	27.1	0.77
101 to 250	25.7	31.4	0.82
251 to 500	31.9	38.4	0.83
501+	36.4	50.7	0.72
Internal medicine			
0 to 50	22.6	35.5	0.64
51 to 100	31.5	30.0	1.05
101 to 250	27.6	33.6	0.82
251 to 500	29.4	38.1	0.77
501+	37.1	46.3	0.80
Orthopedic surgery			
0 to 50	23.4	32.9	0.71
51 to 100	23.5	30.8	0.76
101 to 250	25.3	32.0	0.79
251 to 500	26.2	33.1	0.79
501+	28.2	34.8	0.81

Source: GAO analysis of CMS data.

Notes: We analyzed 100 percent of Medicare Part B claims data and counted physical therapy (PT) services based on the number of PT Healthcare Common Procedure Coding System (HCPCS) services on each claim that Medicare covered in a physician office, PT clinic, outpatient hospital department, skilled nursing facility, comprehensive outpatient rehabilitation facility, rehabilitation agency, or home health agency. For this analysis, we considered providers as self-referring if they self-referred at least one PT service during 2010 and as non-self-referring if they referred at least one PT service to a professional office during 2010 and none of their referrals were self-referred.

To identify providers as practicing in urban areas, we used urban-rural commuting area codes, which are a Census-tract-based classification scheme. In 2010, there were 4,869 self-referring providers in family practice, 4,367 in internal medicine, and 6,458 in orthopedic surgery in urban areas. There were 35,977 non-self-referring providers in family practice, 39,981 in internal medicine, and 11,463 in orthopedic surgery in urban areas.

[a]The Medicare beneficiary practice size for each provider refers to the number of unique beneficiaries that received at least one service in a professional office from that provider during 2010 for any medical condition that was covered by Medicare. Some referring providers had a beneficiary practice size of zero because they treated all their Medicare fee-for-service (FFS) beneficiaries in a setting other than a professional office (such as a hospital outpatient department).

[b]The relative rate of self-referring providers refers to the factor by which the average number of services referred by self-referring providers is different from the average number of services referred by non-self-referring providers. For example, if the relative rate of self-referring providers is equal to 2, it would mean that, on average, self-referring providers referred 2 times as many PT services as did non-self-referring providers.

Table 6. Average Number of Physical Therapy Services Received per Medicare Beneficiary in Rural Areas, by Provider Referral Status, Selected Specialty, and Beneficiary Practice Size in 2010

Provider specialty and Medicare beneficiary practice size[a]	Rural self-referring providers	Rural non-self-referring providers	Relative rate of self-referring providers[b]
Family practice			
0 to 50	32.6	34.9	0.93
51 to 100	18.3	37.5	0.49
101 to 250	20.7	34.7	0.60
251 to 500	28.1	39.8	0.71
501+	39.5	47.1	0.84
Internal medicine			
0 to 50	18.9	43.2	0.44
51 to 100	22.1	38.5	0.57
101 to 250	27.8	34.0	0.82
251 to 500	24.3	36.3	0.67
501+	31.1	43.9	0.71
Orthopedic surgery			
0 to 50	17.3	27.0	0.64
51 to 100	18.7	26.8	0.70
101 to 250	19.6	28.1	0.70
251 to 500	23.3	28.6	0.81
501+	24.2	31.4	0.77

Source: GAO analysis of CMS data.

Notes: We analyzed 100 percent of Medicare Part B claims data and counted physical therapy (PT) services based on the number of PT Healthcare Common Procedure Coding System (HCPCS) services on each claim that Medicare covered in a physician office, PT clinic, outpatient hospital department, skilled nursing facility, comprehensive outpatient rehabilitation facility, rehabilitation agency, or home health agency. We considered providers as self-referring if they self-referred at least one PT service during 2010 and non-self-referring if they referred at least one PT service to a professional office during 2010 and none of their referrals were self-referred. To identify providers as practicing in rural areas, we used urban-rural commuting area codes, which are a Census-tract-based classification scheme. In 2010, there were 964 self-referring providers in family practice, 452 in internal medicine, and 596 in orthopedic surgery in rural areas. There were 11,492 non-self-referring providers in family practice, 5,584 in internal medicine, and 2,327 in orthopedic surgery in rural areas.

[a]The Medicare beneficiary practice size for each provider refers to the number of unique beneficiaries that received at least one service in a professional office from that provider during 2010 for any medical condition that was covered by Medicare. Some referring providers had a beneficiary practice size of zero because they treated all their Medicare fee-for-service (FFS) beneficiaries in a setting other than a professional office (such as a hospital outpatient department).

[b]The relative rate of self-referring providers refers to the factor by which the average number of services referred by self-referring providers is different from the average number of services referred by non-self-referring providers. For example, if the relative rate of self-referring providers is equal to 2, it would mean that, on average, self-referring providers referred 2 times as many PT services as did non-self-referring providers.

While self-referring providers generally referred more beneficiaries during 2010, beneficiaries referred by self-referring providers in family practice, internal medicine, and orthopedic surgery received fewer PT services, on average, compared with beneficiaries referred by non-self-referring providers.[26] For example, in urban areas, beneficiaries referred by self-referring family practice providers received 12 to 28 percent fewer PT services, on average, compared with beneficiaries referred by non-selfreferring family practice providers, depending on the beneficiary practice size category (see table 5).

In rural areas, beneficiaries referred by self-referring providers in family practice, internal medicine, and orthopedic surgery received fewer PT services, on average, than their non-self-referring counterparts in every practice size category (see table 6).

Observed differences between self-referring and non-self-referring providers within each specialty in the number of PT services referred are not likely due to differences in the overall health status of the beneficiaries they referred. We found that self-referring and non-self-referring providers referred beneficiaries who were similar with respect to their average Medicare risk scores[27] and disability status (see table 7). For example, self-referring and non-self-referring family practice providers referred beneficiaries whose average estimated cost to Medicare in 2010 was about 30 percent higher than for the average FFS beneficiary (31 and 33 percent higher, respectively).

Some of the differences between self-referring and non-self-referring providers in the number of PT referrals may be due to differences in the severity or type of medical conditions of the beneficiaries that they referred for PT treatment. Although data on the severity of beneficiaries' medical conditions requiring PT treatment were not available for our study period, we found some differences in the extent to which self-referring and non-self-referring providers referred beneficiaries for selected diagnoses (see table 8). For example, self-referring family practice, internal medicine, and orthopedic surgery providers were more likely to refer beneficiaries who were treated for spine conditions. Non-selfreferring providers in these specialties were more likely to refer beneficiaries who were treated for neurologic conditions or rehabilitation.

Table 7. Selected Characteristics of Medicare Beneficiaries Referred for Physical Therapy Services by Self-Referring and Non-Self-Referring Providers in Selected Specialties, 2010

Beneficiary characteristics, average	Family practice		Internal medicine		Orthopedic surgery	
	Self-referring provider	Non-self-referring provider	Self-referring provider	Non-self-referring provider	Self-referring provider	Non-self-referring provider
Normalized risk score[a]	1.31	1.33	1.45	1.47	1.06	1.07
Percentage age 85 or older	15%	20%	17%	24%	6%	6%
Percentage disabled	18%	16%	13%	11%	15%	17%

Source: GAO analysis of CMS data.

Note: We considered providers to be self-referring if they self-referred at least one physical therapy (PT) service during 2010 and non-self-referring if they referred at least one PT service to a professional office during 2010 and none of their referrals were self-referred.

[a]A beneficiary's risk score is a proxy for health status and is equivalent to the ratio of expected Medicare payments for that beneficiary under Medicare fee-for-service (FFS) relative to the average Medicare payments for all Medicare FFS beneficiaries. The risk scores are normalized using the FFS normalization factor of 1.041 for 2010 that CMS used. Normalization keeps the average FFS risk score constant at 1.0 over time.

Table 8. Percentage of Medicare Beneficiaries Referred for Physical Therapy Services by Self-Referring and Non-SelfReferring Providers in Selected Specialties by Diagnostic Category, 2010

Beneficiary diagnostic category, average[a]	Family practice		Internal medicine		Orthopedic surgery	
	Self-referring provider	Non-self-referring provider	Self-referring provider	Non-self-referring provider	Self-referring provider	Non-self-referring provider
Arthritis	53	56	50	55	69	70
Spine	39	30	40	30	21	19
Sprains	6	4	4	4	7	7
Fractures	3	3	2	4	10	11
Neurologic	17	26	18	28	6	7
Rehabilitation	23	33	23	32	20	29
Other diagnoses	15	24	16	26	4	6

Source: GAO analysis of CMS data.

Note: We considered providers to be self-referring if they self-referred at least one physical therapy (PT) service during 2010 and non-self-referring if they referred at least one PT service to a professional office during 2010 and none of their referrals were self-referred.

[a]The diagnostic categories are defined based on groups of related medical diagnosis codes. They are maintained by the U.S. Agency for Healthcare Research and Quality and are referred to as Clinical Classification Software (CCS) codes. Percentages do not add up to 100 because two or more diagnoses may be reported on a single claim.

In addition, we found some differences in the types of PT treatments used by self-referring and non-self-referring providers. For example, during 2010, self-referring providers in family practice and internal medicine were more likely to refer beneficiaries who were treated with ancillary services such as massage therapy and electrical stimulation. In contrast, non-self-referring providers in these specialties were more likely to refer beneficiaries who were treated with gait training and therapeutic activities (see app. II, which presents tables that show the distribution of PT services by provider specialty and self-referral status).

Table 9. Change in Average Number of Medicare Physical Therapy Services Referred for Self-Referring Providers, Non-SelfReferring Providers, and Switchers in Selected Specialties Who Had at Least One Office Referral, 2008 and 2010

Provider specialty	Referral type	Number of providers with at least one office referral	Average 2008 referred services	Average 2010 referred services	Percentag e change, 2008 to 2010	Percentage pointdifference, switchersand non-self-referringproviders
Family practice	Self-referring	3,572	699	798	14.2%	
	Non-self-referring	29,951	547	621	13.7%	
	Switchers	439	582	775	33.2%	19.5%
Internal medicine	Self-referring	3,110	1,039	1,079	3.9%	
	Non-self-referring	30,969	771	863	12.0%	
	Switchers	412	733	951	29.8%	17.8%
	Referral type	Number of providers with at least one office referral	Average 2008 referred services	Average 2010 referred services	Percentag e change, 2008 to 2010	Percentage pointdifference, switchersand non-self-referringproviders
Orthopedic surgery	Self-referring	5,523	2,146	2,281	6.3%	
	Non-self-referring	10,573	1,716	1,777	3.6%	
	Switchers	514	1,767	1,896	7.3%	3.7%

Source: GAO analysis of CMS data.

Notes: We analyzed 100 percent of Medicare Part B claims data and counted physical therapy (PT) services based on the number of PT Healthcare Common Procedure Coding System (HCPCS) services on each claim that Medicare covered in a physician office, PT clinic, outpatient hospital department, skilled nursing facility, comprehensive outpatient rehabilitation facility, rehabilitation agency, or home health agency. We considered providers to be self-referring if they self-referred at least one PT service in 2008, 2009, and 2010 and non-self-referring if they referred at least one PT service to a professional office in 2008, 2009, and 2010 and none of their referrals were self-referred. We defined switchers as providers who were non-self-referring in 2008 and self-referring in 2009 and 2010. Switchers may have started to self-refer in 2009 by hiring PT provider(s) or joining a group practice that self-referred.

Providers' Referrals for PT Services Increased the Year After They Began to Self-Refer

PT service referrals for providers in family practice, internal medicine, and orthopedic surgery increased the year after they began to self-refer at a higher rate relative to non-self-referring providers of the same specialty. We compared the average number of PT service referrals made by providers that began self-referring beneficiaries for PT services in 2009 and continued doing so in 2010 ("switchers") with the average number of service referrals made by providers who were non-self-referring between 2008 and 2010. The percentage increase in average PT service referrals for switchers between 2008 and 2010 ranged from approximately 7 percent for orthopedic surgeons to 33 percent for family practice providers. In contrast, the percentage increase in the average number of PT service referrals for non-self-referring providers during this time was lower, ranging from approximately 4 percent for orthopedic surgeons to 14 percent for family practice providers (see table 9). The percentage point difference in the number of PT services referred between switchers and non-self-referring providers was higher for family practice and internal medicine providers (approximately 20 percent and 18 percent, respectively) and lower for orthopedic surgeons (approximately 4 percent). This is consistent with our earlier finding that self-referring family practice and internal medicine providers tended to have higher relative referral rates, on average, than their non-self-referring counterparts in 2010, while this effect was much more limited for orthopedic surgeons.

CONCLUSION

By improving patients' physical functioning, strength, or mobility, PT treatment offers many Medicare beneficiaries the opportunity to restore function that they may have lost due to illness or injury. Proponents of PT self-referral contend that it has the potential to improve coordination of care and provide convenient access to PT services. Our review indicates that PT service use and expenditures grew considerably from 2004 to 2010, despite a slight decrease in the total number of FFS beneficiaries over this period. The primary driver of this growth was growth in non-selfreferred services. These results differ from our prior work on self-referral of other Medicare services—namely, advanced imaging, anatomic pathology, and intensity-modulated radiation therapy—in which we reported that self-referred services and expenditures grew faster than non-self-referred services and expenditures. One potential reason for this difference is that non-self-referred PT services can be performed by providers who can directly influence the amount, duration, and frequency of PT services through the written plan of care required by Medicare. In contrast, non-self-referred services we examined for our prior work tend to be performed by providers who have more limited ability to generate additional services or referrals; for example, radiologists generally do not have the discretion to order more imaging services or more intense imaging procedures.

Regardless, substantial growth in PT services raises concerns about higher costs for Medicare and beneficiaries. Although this growth is primarily due to non-self-referred services, we found notable differences between non-self-referring and self-referring providers. For example, we found that average PT service referrals, average PT beneficiary referrals, and average PT services per beneficiary differed based on whether the providers self-referred; further, PT service referrals increased the year after a provider began to self-refer at a higher relative rate to non-selfreferring providers of the same specialty. Better understanding the differences in referral patterns between self-referring and non-selfreferring providers may provide useful information to help manage growth in PT services. In 2013, CMS began collecting additional information on beneficiary functional status on all PT claims. These data may help CMS to better assess the appropriateness and effectiveness of PT treatment provided by both self-referring and non-self-referring providers.

AGENCY AND THIRD-PARTY COMMENTS AND OUR EVALUATION

We provided a draft of this report to HHS, which oversees CMS, for comment. HHS thanked GAO for the opportunity to review the draft and stated that it had no comments. We obtained written comments from four professional associations selected because they represent an array of stakeholders with specific involvement in referring PT services: the American Academy of Family Physicians (AAFP), which represents physicians in family practice; the American Academy of Orthopaedic Surgeons (AAOS), which represents orthopedic surgeons; the American College of Physicians (ACP), which represents physicians in internal medicine; and the American Physical Therapy Association (APTA), which represents physical therapists. The following sections contain a summary of these organizations' comments on our methodology and findings and our response to these comments. We incorporated any technical comments provided where appropriate.

American Academy of Family Physicians

AAFP appreciated the opportunity to review the draft report, but expressed a concern that our methodology to define self-referring providers as those with at least one self-referred PT service to a professional office may skew our results if the majority of the PT services referred by several self-referring providers were not self-referred. We applied this same threshold in our previous work on self-referral, as it is a conservative method for determining providers' self-referral status. Furthermore, we examined the distribution of self-referred PT services to professional offices during 2010 and found that providers who self-refer tended to self-refer a majority of the PT services utilized.

AAFP also provided some context for our findings, noting that some factors may account for our finding that overall spending for PT services increased. For example, AAFP stated that health insurers have encouraged providers to use imaging procedures, surgery for back pain, and medications that manage pain (such as opioids) less frequently. According to AAFP, some providers may be choosing to use less imaging and treat fewer patients with surgery or opioids and instead manage these patients by referring them for PT services. AAFP considers PT a more cost-effective yet less invasive way to treat patients. In addition, AAFP believes that one possible explanation for GAO's finding that self-referring providers referred fewer PT services per beneficiary, on average, than non-self-referring providers, is that providers who self-refer are likely to fully understand the variety of services that are available in the PT facility for which they have an ownership interest.

American Academy of Orthopaedic Surgeons

AAOS appreciated the opportunity to review the draft report and was pleased to see that the data showed that self-referring orthopedic practices generally self-referred the smallest number of PT services per beneficiary on average when compared to other specialty groups in our study. However, AAOS stated that it did not believe there was a rationale for examining “switchers”—providers who became self-referrers during our period of study—because we found that self-referring providers referred fewer services per beneficiary on average. We conducted an analysis of switchers to isolate the effects of self-referral, using a methodology similar to our previous reports on self-referral in Medicare. As noted in the draft report, the average number of PT service referrals made by providers that began self-referring beneficiaries for PT services in 2009 increased at a higher rate relative to non-self-referring providers of the same specialty during our period of study. Specifically, among these “switchers,” the percentage increase in average PT service referrals between 2008 and 2010 was approximately 4 percentage points higher for orthopedic surgeons, 18 percentage points higher for internal medicine providers, and 20 percentage points higher for family practice providers.

AAOS made two additional points for our consideration. First, AAOS noted that self-referring orthopedic surgeons may also refer some services outside of their practice. Our analyses provided a picture of self-referral at both the service and provider levels. Specifically, for our analysis of trends between 2004 and 2010 in the utilization of and expenditures for self-referred and non-self-referred services, we examined each PT service to determine if it was self-referred or not by matching the Taxpayer Identification Number (TIN) on the claim with a crosswalk of the TINs associated with each provider submitting claims. This method allowed us to examine utilization and spending for each PT service—self-referred and non-self-referred. For our analysis of self-referring providers, as we note in the draft report, we considered a provider to be non-self-referring if the provider referred at least one beneficiary for a PT service in a professional office and did not self-refer any PT services. Conversely, we considered a provider to be self-referring if the provider self-referred at least one beneficiary for a PT service that was provided in a professional office during our period of study. Second, AAOS noted that nine states have changed their laws governing self-referral to PT services during the study period and that this may impact our results. We agree that this may impact our results, but examining state laws governing self-referral were outside the scope of this report.

American College of Physicians

ACP stated that a major conclusion of our report, that the primary driver of growth in Medicare expenditures and utilization of PT services was due to non-self-referred PT services, differs from our prior work on self-referral for advanced imaging, anatomic pathology, and intensity-modulated radiation therapy services. According to ACP, this finding demonstrates the complex effects of self-referral on Medicare utilization and expenditures, which may be influenced by type of service as well as the other variables outlined in this report, such as provider specialty, geographic location, and Medicare beneficiary practice size. ACP also stated that the primary payment model can also affect the relationship between self-referral, expenditures, and utilization. For example, practices that participate in Medicare Shared Savings[28] and other value-based payment models likely refer in a different manner than those paid predominantly through the traditional Medicare FFS payment system. While we agree that different payment models could affect physicians' referral patterns, such payment models generally had not been implemented by Medicare at the time of our study. ACP also stated that it is important to consider the extent to which services are ordered on the basis of recognized appropriate use criteria. However, using appropriate use criteria can involve assessing the severity of symptoms in order to determine the appropriate course of treatment, and data on severity were not available at the time of our study. ACP believes that self-referral alone cannot explain expenditure growth differences and that, if utilized appropriately, self-referral allows for increased quality oversight by ordering physicians, better care coordination, and the potential for the provision of lower-cost care compared to alternative settings, such as hospitals.

American Physical Therapy Association

APTA acknowledged the thoroughness of the draft report and appreciated our comprehensive analysis. According to APTA, our findings that self-referring providers referred more beneficiaries for PT services, and that PT referrals for switchers in the three specialties we examined increased relative to non-self-referring providers, are consistent with other studies that found that providers have a financial interest to self-refer. However, APTA also expressed concerns about some of our results. Specifically, APTA noted that patient condition, physical impairments, and comorbidities have a major impact on the amount, duration, and frequency of PT services provided, and without this information it is difficult to draw conclusions about the impact of self-referral arrangements on the frequency of PT services. For example, APTA noted that the frequency of PT use could be attributed to differences in the complexity of the conditions of patients treated by self-referring compared with non-self-referring providers. It also expressed concern that the measures of health status in this report—such as disability status, average risk score, and Clinical Classification Software (CCS) diagnostic categories—are limited in their ability to explain differences in PT frequency. In this report, we state that some of the differences between self-referring and non-self-referring providers in the number of PT referrals may be due to differences in the severity or type of medical conditions of the beneficiaries that they referred for PT treatment. We also acknowledge that data on the severity of beneficiaries' medical conditions requiring PT treatment were not available for our study period. Given the lack of severity data, we examined risk scores, age, and disability status, and described these measures as "overall health status variables," and we present data on beneficiary diagnostic categories without labeling them as measures of severity. We also note that APTA agreed with our conclusion that data CMS began collecting in 2013 may help the agency to better assess the appropriateness and effectiveness of PT treatment for both self-referring and non self-referring providers.

APTA also expressed concerns that including data on PT referrals to facilities, such as outpatient hospitals and skilled nursing facilities, may have affected the results shown in the tables in appendix II of this report, which compare the distribution of Medicare PT services for self-referring and non-self-referring providers. According to APTA, our assumption that all PT services referred to facilities were non-self-referred neglects a significant portion of self-referral arrangements. APTA also stated that because patients in facility settings tend to be more medically complex than patients seen in physician offices, these tables may make an unfair comparison. As we note in the limitations section of this report, we acknowledge that we may have understated the occurrence of certain self-referral arrangements, such as referring physician ownership of hospitals, by assuming that all PT services referred to facilities were nonself-referred. For example, some providers may have referred beneficiaries for PT services to hospital(s) in which they had a financial interest in the entire hospital, and, due to data limitations, we did not analyze the extent to which this type of referral may have occurred.

James Cosgrove
Director, Health Care

APPENDIX I: SCOPE AND METHODOLOGY

This appendix describes the scope and methodology used to analyze our study objectives: (1) trends in the number of and expenditures for self-referred and non-self-referred Medicare physical therapy (PT) services from 2004 through 2010, and (2) how provision of these services differs among providers on the basis of whether they self-refer. For both objectives, we used 100 percent of fee-for-service (FFS) claims from the Medicare Part B Carrier file, which contains final action Medicare Part B claims for noninstitutional providers, such as physicians. For the second objective, we also used 100 percent of FFS claims from the Medicare Outpatient Claims file, which includes final action Medicare Part B claims for five types of facilities that also provide PT services: outpatient hospitals, skilled nursing facilities, comprehensive outpatient rehabilitation facilities, rehabilitation agencies, and home health agencies.

Each Medicare claim contains data for one or more services for a particular beneficiary. Each service is identified on a claim by its Healthcare Common Procedure Coding System (HCPCS) code, which the Centers for Medicare & Medicaid Services (CMS) assigns to products, supplies, and services for billing purposes. To identify all PT services covered by Medicare, we used outpatient therapy HCPCS codes published in the Federal Register and in CMS's Annual Therapy Update to identify the universe of outpatient therapy HCPCS codes in use from 2004 through 2010. We then used the HCPCS code claim modifier (for Carrier file claims) and Revenue Center code (for Outpatient file claims) to distinguish PT services from occupational therapy or speech-language pathology services. Because there is no indicator or flag on the claim that identifies whether services were self-referred or non-self-referred, we developed a claims-based methodology to identify services as either self-referred or non-self-referred. Specifically, we classified services as self-referred if the provider that referred the beneficiary for a PT service and the provider that performed the PT service were identical or had a financial relationship.[1] To determine providers' financial relationships, we used the Taxpayer Identification Number (TIN), which is either the Social Security Number or Employer Identification Number that an individual or organization uses to report tax information to the Internal Revenue Service. A TIN could be that of the provider, the provider's employer, or another entity to which the provider reassigns payment.[2] There may be one or multiple TINs for a medical group practice depending on the organizational structure of the practice.[3] To identify the associated TINs for the referring and performing providers, we created a crosswalk of the performing provider's unique physician identification number, or national provider identifier (NPI), to the TIN that appeared on the claim and used that to assign TINs to the referring and performing providers.[4]

To describe the trends in the number of and expenditures for self-referred PT services from 2004 through 2010, we used the 100 percent Medicare Part B Carrier file for each year to calculate utilization and expenditures for self-referred and non-self-referred PT services. We focused on PT referrals to professional offices, such as physician offices or PT clinics, because the financial incentive for providers to self-refer is most direct when the service is performed in a professional office. To calculate utilization, we counted the number of PT HCPCS codes. We also calculated the average number of 15-minute units provided per PT service.[5] To calculate expenditures, we used the allowed charges variable, which includes payments by Medicare and the beneficiary.

To determine the extent to which the provision of PT services differs for providers who self-refer when compared with other providers, we classified providers based on the type of referrals they made each year between 2008 and 2010. Specifically, we classified providers as self-referring during a year if they self-referred at least one beneficiary for a PT service that was provided in a professional office. We classified providers as non-self-referring if they referred at least one beneficiary for a PT service in a professional office and did not self-refer any PT services. [6] We then performed two separate analyses. For the first analysis, we compared the number of referrals made for PT services by self-referring providers and non-self-referring providers in 2010. Because the amount, frequency, and duration of PT services may vary for each beneficiary, we examined three PT referral measures for each referring provider: total number of PT services referred, total number of beneficiary referrals to an office or facility, and average number of PT services received by each beneficiary referred. We assumed that all beneficiaries referred to facilities were provided non-self-referred PT services.[7] We compared the number of PT referrals made by self-referring and non-self-referring providers in 2010, disaggregated by selected provider specialty, Medicare beneficiary practice size, and geography (i.e., urban or rural provider location). We identified providers' specialties on the basis of the specialties listed on the claims. We report results for three physician specialties that referred nearly 75 percent of PT services during 2010 that had a unique referring provider identification number—family practice (20 percent), internal medicine (26 percent), and orthopedic surgery (28 percent).[8] We calculated beneficiary practice size by computing the number of unique Medicare FFS beneficiaries that providers treated in a professional office in 2010 for any medical condition covered by Medicare. We defined urban settings as metropolitan statistical areas, a geographic entity defined by the Office of Management and Budget as a core urban area of 50,000 or more population. We used rural-urban commuting area codes—a Census tract-based classification scheme that utilizes the standard Bureau of Census Urbanized Area and Urban Cluster definitions in combination with work commuting information to characterize all of the nation's Census tracts regarding their rural and urban status—to identify providers as practicing in metropolitan statistical areas.[9] We considered all other settings to be rural.[10]

In addition, we examined the extent to which the characteristics of the beneficiaries referred by self-referring and non-self-referring providers differed. We used CMS's risk score file to identify each beneficiary's risk score, age (specifically, whether the beneficiary was age 85 or older), and disability status.[11] The risk score is an estimate of each beneficiary's overall health status. It is the ratio of expected Medicare payments for that beneficiary under Medicare FFS relative to the average health care payments for all Medicare FFS beneficiaries.[12] We used the Clinical Classification Software (CCS) categories maintained by the U.S. Agency for Healthcare Research and Quality to identify the diagnostic category for which each beneficiary received PT treatment. The CCS categories are based on International Classification of Diseases, 9th Revision, Clinical Modification (ICD-9-CM), a uniform and standardized diagnostic and procedural coding system. The CCS categories group ICD-9-CM codes into a smaller number of clinically meaningful categories. The CCS diagnostic categories for PT that we used include Arthritis/Other Connective Tissue and Joint Disorders, Fractures/Traumatic Joint Disorders, Neurological, Spine, Sprains/Strains, V codes/Miscellaneous Rehab, and Other PT diagnoses.

For the second analysis, we determined the extent to which the number of PT service referrals made by providers changed after they began to self-refer. Specifically, we identified a group of providers, whom we called "switchers," that were non-self-referring in 2008 and self-referring in 2009 and 2010. We then calculated the change in the number of PT referrals made from 2008 (i.e., the year before the switchers began self-referring) to 2010 (i.e., the year after they began self-referring). We compared the change in the number of referrals made by these providers to the change in the number of referrals made over the same time period by providers who were non-self-referring between 2008 and 2010. Differences in the average number of PT services referred by non-self-referring providers between 2008 and 2010 reflect changes during this period that were not related to self-referral, such as changes in the number of beneficiaries who needed PT services or changes in the severity or types of the medical conditions treated with PT. Differences in the average number of PT services referred by switchers may reflect these changes as well as changes associated with self-referral. The difference in the percentage change in the number of PT services referred by switchers and non-selfreferring providers is an estimate of the change in providers' referrals for PT services that may be associated with self-referral.

Our study has some limitations. First, we may not have identified all self-referred PT services, because CMS uses the referring provider identifier on PT claims to identify the provider who certified the beneficiary's plan of care, and in some cases the referring provider may be different from the certifying provider. In addition, Medicare claims data do not capture all financial relationships between performing and referring providers. Second, we may have understated the occurrence of certain self-referral arrangements, such as referring physician ownership of hospitals, by assuming that all PT services referred to facilities were non-self-referred. Third, our analysis that compares PT diagnostic categories for beneficiaries referred by self-referring and non-self-referring providers is based on data that CMS does not use to determine payment for PT services. Consequently, providers do not have a financial incentive to accurately report diagnostic data for PT services on Medicare claims. Finally, it is outside the scope of this report to examine the medical necessity, clinical appropriateness, or effectiveness of PT services beneficiaries received.

We took several steps to ensure that the data used to produce this report were sufficiently reliable. Specifically, we assessed the reliability of the CMS data we used by interviewing officials responsible for overseeing these data sources, including CMS and Medicare contractor officials. We also reviewed relevant documentation, compared means and frequencies of selected variables with published data, and examined the data for obvious errors, such as missing values and values outside of expected ranges. We determined that the data were sufficiently reliable for the purposes of our study, as they are used by the Medicare program as a record of payments to health care providers. As such, they are subject to routine CMS scrutiny.

We conducted this performance audit from February 2012 through April 2014 in accordance with generally accepted government auditing standards. Those standards require that we plan and perform the audit to obtain sufficient, appropriate evidence to provide a reasonable basis for our findings and conclusions based on our audit objectives. We believe that the evidence obtained provides a reasonable basis for our findings and conclusions based on our audit objectives.

APPENDIX II: DISTRIBUTION OF MEDICARE PHYSICAL THERAPY SERVICES FOR SELF-REFERRING AND NON-SELF-REFERRING PROVIDERS, 2010

Table 10. Distribution of Physical Therapy Services for Self-Referring and Non-Self-Referring Family Practice Providers, 2010

	Percentage of all PT services		
Physical therapy (PT) service[a]	Self-referring family practice providers	Non-self-referring family practice providers	Percentage point difference
Electrical stimulation (HCPCS 97032)	3.5	1.2	2.3
Electrical stimulation, other than wound (HCPCS G0283)	7.3	6.2	1.1
Gait training therapy (HCPCS 97116)	7.5	12.0	-4.5
Manual therapy (HCPCS 97140)	13.1	10.7	2.4
Massage therapy (HCPCS 97124)	3.2	0.5	2.7
Neuromuscular reeducation (HCPCS 97112)	10.4	9.8	0.6
Physical therapy evaluation (HCPCS 97001)	3.1	3.5	-0.4
Therapeutic activities (HCPCS 97530)	10.0	12.7	-2.7
Therapeutic exercises (HCPCS 97110)	30.3	33.7	-3.4
Ultrasound therapy (HCPCS 97035)	5.6	4.2	1.4
Subtotal	94.0	94.5	—
All other PT services	6.0	5.5	—
Total	100	100	—

Source: GAO analysis of CMS data.

Note: We analyzed 100 percent of Medicare Part B claims data and counted PT services based on the number of PT Healthcare Common Procedure Coding System (HCPCS) services on each claim that Medicare covered in a physician office, PT clinic, outpatient hospital department, skilled nursing facility, comprehensive outpatient rehabilitation facility, rehabilitation agency, or home health agency.

[a]We considered providers to be self-referring if they self-referred at least one PT service during 2010, and non-self-referring if they referred at least one PT service to a professional office during 2010 and none of their referrals were self-referred.

Table 11. Distribution of Medicare Physical Therapy Services for Self-Referring and Non-Self-Referring Internal Medicine Providers, 2010

	Percentage of all PT services		
Physical therapy (PT) service[a]	Self-referring internal medicine providers	Non-self-referring internal medicine providers	Percentage point difference
Electrical stimulation (HCPCS 97032)	3.9	1.3	2.6
Electrical stimulation, other than wound (HCPCS G0283)	7.8	5.5	2.3
Gait training therapy (HCPCS 97116)	6.9	12.3	-5.4
Manual therapy (HCPCS 97140)	13.8	10.6	3.2
Massage therapy (HCPCS 97124)	2.9	0.6	2.3
Neuromuscular reeducation (HCPCS 97112)	9.3	10.9	-1.6
Physical therapy evaluation (HCPCS 97001)	2.8	3.3	-0.5
Therapeutic activities (HCPCS 97530)	10.6	13.0	-2.4
Therapeutic exercises (HCPCS 97110)	30.1	33.7	-3.6
Ultrasound therapy (HCPCS 97035)	6.6	3.6	3.0
Subtotal	94.7	94.8	—
All other PT services	5.3	5.2	—
Total	100	100	—

Source: GAO analysis of CMS data.

Note: We analyzed 100 percent of Medicare Part B claims data and counted PT services based on the number of PT Healthcare Common Procedure Coding System (HCPCS) services on each claim that Medicare covered in a physician office, PT clinic, outpatient hospital department, skilled nursing facility, comprehensive outpatient rehabilitation facility, rehabilitation agency, or home health agency.

[a]We considered providers to be self-referring if they self-referred at least one PT service during 2010, and non-self-referring if they referred at least one PT service to a professional office during 2010 and none of their referrals were self-referred.

Table 12. Distribution of Medicare Physical Therapy Services for Self-Referring and Non-Self-Referring Orthopedic Surgery Providers, 2010

	Percentage of all physical therapy services		
Physical therapy (PT) service[a]	Self-referring orthopedic surgery providers	Non-self-referring orthopedic surgery providers	Percentage point difference
Electrical stimulation (HCPCS 97032)	1.4	1.6	-0.2
Electrical stimulation, other than wound (HCPCS G0283)	10.5	10.4	0.1
Gait training therapy (HCPCS 97116)	1.4	1.5	-0.1

Table 12. (Continued)

Physical therapy (PT) service[a]	Percentage of all physical therapy services		
	Self-referring orthopedic surgery providers	Non-self-referring orthopedic surgery providers	Percentage point difference
Manual therapy (HCPCS 97140)	20.3	21.0	-0.7
Massage therapy (HCPCS 97124)	0.4	0.4	0.0
Neuromuscular reeducation (HCPCS 97112)	5.2	5.7	-0.5
Physical therapy evaluation (HCPCS 97001)	4.0	3.6	0.4
Therapeutic activities (HCPCS 97530)	5.1	5.5	-0.4
Therapeutic exercises (HCPCS 97110)	40.5	39.3	1.2
Ultrasound therapy (HCPCS 97035)	4.6	4.7	-0.1
Subtotal	93.4	93.7	—
All other PT services	6.6	6.3	—
Total	100	100	—

Source: GAO analysis of CMS data.

Note: We analyzed 100 percent of Medicare Part B claims data and counted PT services based on the number of PT Healthcare Common Procedure Coding System (HCPCS) services on each claim that Medicare covered in a physician office, PT clinic, outpatient hospital department, skilled nursing facility, comprehensive outpatient rehabilitation facility, rehabilitation agency, or home health agency.

[a]We considered providers to be self-referring if they self-referred at least one PT service during 2010, and non-self-referring if they referred at least one PT service to a professional office during 2010 and none of their referrals were self-referred.

APPENDIX III: PROVIDERS WHO REFERRED MEDICARE PHYSICAL THERAPY SERVICES, BY SELECTED CHARACTERISTICS, 2010

Table 13. Providers in Urban Areas Who Referred Medicare Physical Therapy Services, by Provider Referral Status, Selected Specialty, and Beneficiary Practice Size in 2010

Provider specialty and Medicare beneficiary practice size[a]	Urban self-referring providers	Urban non-self-referring providers
Family practice		
0 to 50	0.2%	3.2%
51 to 100	0.3%	1.9%
101 to 250	0.9%	6.5%
251 to 500	0.8%	5.2%
501+	0.4%	1.9%
Internal medicine		
0 to 50	0.1%	3.0%

Provider specialty and Medicare beneficiary practice sizea	Urban self-referring providers	Urban non-self-referring providers
51 to 100	0.1%	1.3%
101 to 250	0.6%	5.0%
251 to 500	0.8%	6.7%
501+	0.7%	4.9%
Orthopedic surgery		
0 to 50	0.1%	1.1%
51 to 100	0.1%	0.5%
101 to 250	0.8%	1.7%
251 to 500	1.4%	1.9%
501+	0.9%	0.7%
All practice sizes for the three specialties		
Percentage of urban referring providers	8.1%	45.3%
Number of urban referring providers	15,694	87,421

Source: GAO analysis of CMS data.

Notes: We analyzed 100 percent of Medicare Part B claims data for physical therapy (PT) services that Medicare covered in a physician office, PT clinic, outpatient hospital department, skilled nursing facility, comprehensive outpatient rehabilitation facility, rehabilitation agency, or home health agency. We considered providers to be self-referring if they self-referred at least one PT service during 2010 and non-self-referring if they referred at least one PT service to a professional office during 2010 and none of their referrals were self-referred. To identify providers as practicing in urban areas, we used urban-rural commuting area codes, which are a Census-tract-based classification scheme. In 2010, there were 4,869 self-referring providers in family practice, 4,367 in internal medicine, and 6,458 in orthopedic surgery in urban areas. There were 35,977 non-self-referring providers in family practice, 39,981 in internal medicine, and 11,463 in orthopedic surgery in urban areas. In 2010, there were 192,809 providers in urban areas from all specialties who referred PT services.

[a]The Medicare beneficiary practice size for each provider refers to the number of unique Medicare fee-for-service (FFS) beneficiaries that received at least one service in a professional office from that provider during 2010 for any medical condition that was covered by Medicare. Some referring providers had a beneficiary practice size of zero because they treated all their Medicare FFS beneficiaries in a setting other than a professional office (such as a hospital outpatient department).

Table 14. Providers in Rural Areas who Referred Medicare Physical Therapy Services, by Provider Referral Status, Selected Specialty, and Beneficiary Practice Size in 2010

Provider specialty and Medicare beneficiary practice size[a]	Rural self-referring providers	Rural non-selfreferring providers
Family practice		
0 to 50	0.1%	4.8%
51 to 100	0.1%	2.4%
101 to 250	0.7%	8.0%
251 to 500	1.1%	10.9%
501+	0.7%	6.1%
Internal medicine		
0 to 50	0.0%[b]	1.5%
51 to 100	0.0%[b]	0.5%
101 to 250	0.2%	2.1%

Table 14. (Continueda0

Provider specialty and Medicare beneficiary practice sizea	Rural self-referring providers	Rural non-selfreferring providers
251 to 500	0.4%	4.6%
501+	0.6%	7.1%
Orthopedic surgery		
0 to 50	0.0%[b]	0.7%
51 to 100	0.0%[b]	0.3%
101 to 250	0.3%	1.5%
251 to 500	0.8%	2.6%
501+	0.6%	1.4%
All practice sizes for the three specialties		
Percentage of rural referring providers	5.7%	54.6%
Number of rural referring providers	2,012	19,403

Source: GAO analysis of CMS data.

Notes: We analyzed 100 percent of Medicare Part B claims data for physical therapy (PT) services that Medicare covered in a physician office, PT clinic, outpatient hospital department, skilled nursing facility, comprehensive outpatient rehabilitation facility, rehabilitation agency, or home health agency. We considered providers to be self-referring if they self-referred at least one PT service during 2010 and non-self-referring if they referred at least one PT service to a professional office during 2010 and none of their referrals were self-referred. To identify providers as practicing in rural areas, we used urban-rural commuting area codes, which are a Census-tract-based classification scheme. In 2010, there were 964 self-referring providers in family practice, 452 in internal medicine, and 596 in orthopedic surgery in rural areas. There were 11,492 non-self-referring providers in family practice, 5.584 in internal medicine, and 2,327 in orthopedic surgery in rural areas. In 2010, there were 35,546 providers in rural areas from all specialties who referred PT services.

[a]The Medicare beneficiary practice size for each provider refers to the number of unique Medicare fee-for-service (FFS) beneficiaries that received at least one service in a professional office from that provider during 2010 for any medical condition that was covered by Medicare. Some referring providers had a beneficiary practice size of zero because they treated all their Medicare FFS beneficiaries in a setting other than a professional office (such as a hospital outpatient department).

[b]Values given as 0.0 percent are values less than 0.05 percent, rounded to zero.

End Notes

[1] Pub. L. No. 105-33, § 4541, 111 Stat. 251, 454. BBA established a combined $1,500 cap for PT and speech-language pathology for calendar year 1999. The amount of the therapy caps is calculated annually to account for increases in the Medicare economic index, and has increased to $1,920 in 2014 for PT and speech-language pathology services combined. Since BBA, therapy caps were in effect only in 1999 and in part of 2003; in other years, Congress imposed temporary moratoria on the caps in response to concerns that patients with an extensive need for outpatient therapy services might be adversely affected by the caps. See, for example, Medicare, Medicaid, and SCHIP Balanced Budget Refinement Act of 1999, Pub. L. No. 106-113, App. F, § 221(a), 113 Stat. 1501, 1501A351; Medicare, Medicaid, and SCHIP Benefits Improvement and Protection Act of 2000, Pub. L. No. 106-554, App. F, § 421(a), 114, Stat. 2763, 2763A-516; Medicare Prescription Drug, Improvement, and Modernization Act of 2003 (MMA), Pub. L. No. 108-173, § 624(a), 117 Stat. 2066, 2317.

[2] Pub. L. No. 112-96, § 3005(g), 126 Stat. 156, 189. The Middle Class Tax Relief and Job Creation Act of 2012 made several changes affecting the processing of claims for outpatient therapy services. For example, the act

required CMS to begin conducting manual medical reviews of requests for exceptions for outpatient therapy claims over an annual threshold of $3,700 for services provided on or after October 1, 2012 and required that the national provider identification number of the physician who certifies the plan of care be included on Medicare claims for outpatient therapy services, including PT.

[3] For example, a provider may refer patients to a physical therapist who is employed by the provider or the provider's group practice.

[4] Compliance with the physician self-referral law, commonly known as the Stark Law, is outside the scope of this report. The Stark Law prohibits physicians from making referrals for certain designated health services paid for by Medicare to entities with which the physicians or immediate family members have a financial relationship, unless the arrangement complies with a specific exception, such as in-office ancillary services. 42 U.S.C. § 1395nn(b)(2). The requirements of the in-office ancillary services exception are found at 42 C.F.R § 411.355(b)(2013).

[5] For studies by GAO on physician self-referral, see GAO, *Medicare: Higher Use of Advanced Imaging Services by Providers Who Self-Refer Costing Medicare Millions,* GAO-12-966 (Washington, D.C.: Sept. 28, 2012); GAO, *Medicare: Action Needed to Address Higher Use of Anatomic Pathology Services by Providers Who Self-Refer,* GAO-13-445 (Washington, D.C.: June 24, 2013); and GAO, *Medicare: Higher Use of Costly Prostate Cancer Treatment by Providers Who Self-Refer Warrants Scrutiny*, GAO-13-525 (Washington, D.C.: July 19, 2013).

[6] Medicare data from the Carrier file include data from the CMS-1500, which is the standard claim form used by noninstitutional providers, such as physicians' offices and physical therapists' private practices, to bill Medicare. Some of the PT services reported on the CMS-1500 may be provided in patients' homes. We used Healthcare Common Procedure Coding System (HCPCS) codes to identify PT services, and included claims for all office-based PT services that were covered by Medicare.

[7] Providers could have a financial relationship with the same entity if, for example, they are part of the same group practice.

[8] CMS uses the provider shown in the referring provider field to identify the provider who certified the beneficiary's plan of care for PT services. In some cases the certifying provider may be different from the referring provider. In this study we refer to the provider shown in the referring provider field as the referring provider.

[9] Expenditure trends are based on allowed charges from the claims. Allowed charges include the payments made by both the beneficiary and the Medicare program.

[10] All self-referring and non-self-referring providers in this study referred at least one PT service to a professional office, and some may have also referred PT services to a facility setting. We assumed that all PT services referred to a facility setting were non-selfreferred services.

[11] For example, the number of PT services providers refer may increase as their Medicare beneficiary practice size increases. Examining PT referral measures for providers within each subgroup helps to account for provider characteristics that may be associated with the amount of PT referrals and provides a better estimate of how providers' PT referral patterns vary on the basis of whether they self-refer.

[12] During 2010, family practice providers referred approximately 20 percent of PT services with a unique referring provider identifier, internal medicine providers referred 26 percent, and orthopedic surgeons referred 28 percent. We also examined other provider specialties that self-referred PT services, including neurology, podiatry, and physical medicine.

[13] 42 CFR §§ 424.24(c)(1)(iii), 410.61(c). For example, the plan of care for PT services may be documented as "once daily, three times per week, over 6 weeks." CMS, *Medicare Benefit Policy Manual*, Chapter 15, § 220.1.2 (2012).

[14] 42 CFR § 424.24(c)(4)(i).

[15] According to the American Physical Therapy Association, 48 states and the District of Columbia have state laws that allow "direct access" to certain PT services without a physician referral. Michigan and Oklahoma allow PT evaluation without referral, but not treatment. The association estimates that less than 10 percent of patients obtain PT services without a physician referral, and this percentage may vary by state depending on the specific provisions in state direct access laws.

[16] For example, a Medicare claim line with a timed PT HCPCS code and a unit count of "2" means that a beneficiary received two 15-minute increments of that service. Not all PT services are timed. For example, the HCPCS code for PT evaluation is untimed.

[17] We previously reported that self-referred services and expenditures for advanced imaging, anatomic pathology, and intensity-modulated radiation therapy grew faster than non-self-referred services and expenditures. See GAO-12-966, GAO-13-445, and GAO-13-525. One potential reason for this difference is that non-self-

referred PT services can be performed by providers who can directly influence the amount, duration, and frequency of PT services through the written plan of care required by Medicare. In contrast, non-self-referred services we examined for our prior work tend to be performed by providers who have more limited ability to generate additional services or referrals; for example, radiologists generally do not have the discretion to order more imaging services or more intense imaging procedures.

[18] As a result of increased enrollment in Medicare Advantage, the number of Medicare FFS beneficiaries decreased from 2004 to 2010, going from approximately 35.5 million to approximately 35.3 million. The Medicare Advantage program is an alternative to the original Medicare FFS program in which private health insurance plans offer health care coverage to Medicare beneficiaries.

[19] Self-referred PT services per 1,000 FFS beneficiaries changed from approximately 320 to approximately 319 (about -0.3 percent) from 2004 to 2010.

[20] Beginning in January 2006, beneficiaries could exceed the therapy payment caps through an exceptions process. Under an automatic exceptions process, beneficiaries who had qualifying conditions could exceed the therapy caps, while those who were not eligible for the automatic exceptions process could apply for a manual exception if they required services beyond the cap. In 2007, the exceptions process became fully automatic, allowing a provider to certify the medical necessity of therapy services in excess of the cap by adding a modifier to the therapy claim.

[21] On average, self-referred PT services were billed for a slightly shorter period of time than non-self-referred PT services. In 2010, the average number of 15-minute units billed per self-referred PT service was 1.4, or approximately 21 minutes per service; in contrast, the average number of 15-minute units billed per non-self-referred PT service was 1.5, which corresponds to approximately 23 minutes of therapy per service. Further, the average number of 15-minute units associated with each self-referred PT service grew less than 1 percent from 2004 through 2010, while the average number of units associated with each non-self-referred PT service grew 5.7 percent over this period.

[22] We determined Medicare beneficiary practice size on the basis of the number of unique Medicare FFS beneficiaries who received at least one service in a professional office from each provider for any medical condition covered by Medicare. Geographic location refers to the urban or rural location based on designations from the U.S. Census Bureau.

[23] During 2010, a smaller percentage of family practice, internal medicine, and orthopedic surgery providers in rural areas were self-referring compared with their urban counterparts.

[24] We classified referring providers into five beneficiary practice size groups: 0 to 50, 51 to 100, 101 to 250, 251 to 500, and 501 or more beneficiaries. Some referring providers had a beneficiary practice size of zero because they treated all their beneficiaries in a setting other than a professional office (such as a hospital outpatient department).

[25] The relative rate of self-referring providers refers to the factor by which the average number of services referred by self-referring providers is different from the average number of services referred by non-self-referring providers. For example, if the relative rate of self-referring providers is equal to 2, it would mean that, on average, self-referring providers referred 2 times as many PT services as did non-self-referring providers.

[26] A study of PT self-referral using worker's compensation data from California found similar results: self-referring providers initiated PT treatment 2.3 times more often than non-self-referring physicians, but the mean cost per case for PT was lower in the self-referral group (see A. Swedlow, G. Johnson, N. Smithline, and A. Milstein, "Increased Costs and Rates of Use in the California Workers' Compensation System as a Result of Self-Referral by Physicians," *The New England Journal of Medicine*, vol. 327, no. 21 (1992)). Examining why beneficiaries referred by self-referring providers received fewer services, on average, compared with beneficiaries referred by non-self-referring providers was beyond the scope of this study.

[27] CMS calculates a risk score for each Medicare beneficiary, which is the ratio of expected Medicare payments for that beneficiary under Medicare FFS relative to the average health care payments for all Medicare FFS beneficiaries. For example, a beneficiary with a risk score of 1.05 would have expected Medicare payments that were 5 percent greater than the average Medicare FFS beneficiary, who is assigned a risk score of 1.

[28] The Medicare Shared Savings Program is a program that encourages coordination of care under Medicare Parts A and B and promotes accountability for patient populations. Under this program, eligible health systems that achieve savings for Medicare by improving quality and efficiency may receive a share of the savings they generate as financial incentive payments.

End Notes for Appendix I

[1] Although physicians have long been required by Medicare to report a provider identification number on claims for services they performed, they were not required to report a provider identification number for services they referred in the referring or attending provider fields in Medicare Part B outpatient claims until 2012. The Middle Class Tax Relief and Job Creation Act of 2012 required that the identification number of the physician who certified the plan of care be included in Medicare outpatient claims for outpatient therapy services, including PT. PL 112-96, § 3005(c), 126 Stat 188.

[2] Some providers may be associated with TINs with which they or their immediate family members do not have a direct or indirect financial relationship and thus would not have the same incentives as other self-referring providers. We anticipate that relatively few providers in our self-referring group meet this description, but to the extent that they do, it may have limited the differences we found in utilization and expenditure rates between self-referring and non-self-referring providers.

[3] For example, all providers in the same medical group practice may have the same TIN. Alternatively, five medical group practices that belong to the same corporate entity may each have a separate TIN.

[4] The final rule implementing the Health Insurance Portability and Accountability Act established the standard for a unique health identifier for health care providers for use in the health care system and announced the adoption of the NPI as that standard. *HIPAA Administrative Simplification: Standard Unique Health Identifier for Health Care Providers*, 69 Fed. Reg. 3434 (Jan. 23, 2004) (adding a new subpart D to 45 C.F.R. part 162). Performing physicians were required to include their NPI on any claim submitted to Medicare as of May 23, 2008. Prior to implementation of the NPI, Medicare required providers to submit another type of unique provider identifier called the unique physician identification number. Our methodology for identifying self-referred services was similar to the methodology we used for our study of physician self-referral of imaging services. See GAO, *Medicare: Higher Use of Advanced Imaging Services by Providers Who Self-Refer Costing Medicare Millions*, GAO-12-966 (Washington, D.C.: Sept. 28, 2012).

[5] The number of 15-minute service units per PT service is reported for timed PT HCPCS codes. For example, a Medicare claim line with a timed PT HCPCS code and a unit count of "2" means that a beneficiary received two 15-minute increments of that service. Not all PT services are timed. For example, the HCPCS codes for PT evaluation and PT reevaluation are untimed.

[6] We also conducted some analyses with an alternative definition of "non-self-referring provider." Our alternative definition of "non-self-referring provider" included providers who referred at least one beneficiary for a PT service in a professional office *or a facility* and did not self-refer any PT services. This alternative definition included an additional 49,062 providers in family practice, internal medicine, and orthopedic surgery who referred beneficiaries for PT services exclusively to facilities during 2010. With this alternative definition, we computed higher relative rates of self-referral for the average number of Medicare beneficiary referrals for PT services and for the average number of PT services provided per beneficiary (except for family practice providers). We decided to use our original definition of non-self-referring provider because it generally produced more conservative results.

[7] Some providers may refer beneficiaries for PT services to hospital(s) in which they have a financial interest in the entire hospital. We did not analyze the extent to which this type of referral may have occurred.

[8] During 2010, we could not identify a unique referring provider for 8.6 percent of PT services provided in professional offices (because a referring provider identifier was missing) and for 2.6 percent of PT services provided in facilities (because two or more referring providers were reported on the claim).

[9] We considered a location with a rural-urban commuting area code of 1.0, 1.1, 2.0, 2.1, or 3.0 to be a metropolitan statistical area.

[10] If we could not find a provider's zip code on the Medicare claim or in the National Plan and Provider Enumeration System file (which has data on the provider's business address for every provider identification number in the file), then we did not classify the provider as having either an urban or a rural location. We were unable to find zip code data for less than 1 percent of the providers who referred a beneficiary for PT services in a professional office during 2010.

[11] Beneficiaries who are enrolled in Medicare because of disability are under age 65 and have been entitled to Social Security disability benefits for at least 24 months.

[12] For example, a beneficiary with a risk score of 1.05 would have expected Medicare payments that were 5 percent greater than the average Medicare FFS beneficiary, who is assigned a risk score of 1.

In: Physician Self-Referrals
Editor: Louise Hamilton

ISBN: 978-1-63463-444-1

Chapter 2

MEDICARE: HIGHER USE OF COSTLY PROSTATE CANCER TREATMENT BY PROVIDERS WHO SELF-REFER WARRANTS SCRUTINY*

United States Government Accountability Office

WHY GAO DID THIS STUDY

Questions have been raised about selfreferral's role in Medicare Part B expenditures' rapid growth. Self-referral occurs when a provider refers patients to entities in which the provider or the provider's family members have a financial interest. Services that can be self-referred under certain circumstances include IMRT, a common and costly treatment for prostate cancer. GAO was asked to examine Medicare self-referral trends among radiation oncology services. This report examines (1) trends in the number of and expenditures for prostate cancer-related IMRT services provided by self-referring and non-selfreferring provider groups from 2006 through 2010 and (2) how the percentage of prostate cancer patients referred for IMRT may differ on the basis of whether providers self-refer. GAO analyzed Medicare Part B claims and developed a claims-based methodology to identify self-referring groups and providers. GAO also interviewed officials from the Centers for Medicare & Medicaid Services (CMS), which administers Medicare, and other stakeholders.

WHAT GAO RECOMMENDS

Congress should consider directing the Secretary of Health and Human Services, whose agency oversees CMS, to require providers to disclose their financial interests in IMRT to their patients. GAO also recommends that CMS identify and monitor self-referral of IMRT services. HHS disagreed with GAO's recommendation. Given the magnitude of GAO's findings, GAO maintains CMS should identify and monitor self-referral of IMRT services.

* This is an edited, reformatted and augmented version of a United States Government Accountability Office publication, No. GAO-13-525, dated July 2013.

What GAO Found

The number of Medicare prostate cancer–related intensity-modulated radiation therapy (IMRT) services performed by self-referring groups increased rapidly, while declining for non-self-referring groups from 2006 to 2010. Over this period, the number of prostate cancer–related IMRT services performed by self-referring groups increased from about 80,000 to 366,000. Consistent with that growth, expenditures associated with these services and the number of self-referring groups also increased. The growth in services performed by self-referring groups was due entirely to limited-specialty groups—groups comprised of urologists and a small number of other specialties—rather than multispecialty groups.

Providers substantially increased the percentage of their prostate cancer patients they referred for IMRT after they began to self-refer. Providers that began self-referring in 2008 or 2009—referred to as switchers—referred 54 percent of their patients who were diagnosed with prostate cancer in 2009 for IMRT, compared to 37 percent of their patients diagnosed in 2007. In contrast, providers who did not begin to self-refer—that is, non-self-referrers and providers who self-referred the entire period—experienced much smaller changes over the same period. Among all providers who referred a Medicare beneficiary diagnosed with prostate cancer in 2009, those that self-referred were 53 percent more likely to refer their patients for IMRT and less likely to refer them for other treatments, especially a radical prostatectomy or brachytherapy.

Change in the Percentage of Medicare Prostate Cancer Patients Providers Referred for IMRT after a Diagnosis of Prostate Cancer in 2007 or 2009

Type of provider	Percentage of providers' patients referred for IMRT among beneficiaries diagnosed in 2007	Percentage of providers' patients referred for IMRT among beneficiaries diagnosed in 2009	Percentage point change from 2007 to 2009	Percentage moreor less likelyproviders were torefer patients forIMRT in 2009compared to 2007
Switchers	37.0%	54.2%	17.2	46.6%
Non-self-referrers	31.4	33.1	1.7	5.5
Self-referrers	55.7	52.9	-2.8	-5.1

Source: GAO analysis of CMS data.

Note: Switchers did not self-refer in 2006 or 2007 but began to self-refer in either 2008 or 2009. The percentage by which providers were more or less likely to refer patients for IMRT in 2009 compared to 2007 is equivalent to the percentage point change from 2007 to 2009 divided by the percentage of providers' patients referred for IMRT among beneficiaries diagnosed in 2007.

Compared to IMRT, those treatments are less costly and often considered equally appropriate but have different risks and side effects. Factors such as age, geographic location, and patient health did not explain the large differences between self-referring and non-self-referring providers. These analyses suggest that financial incentives for self-referring providers—specifically those in limited specialty groups—were likely a major factor driving the increase in the percentage of prostate cancer patients referred for IMRT. Medicare providers are generally not required to disclose that they self-refer IMRT services, and the Department of Health and Human Services (HHS) lacks the authority to establish such a requirement. Thus, beneficiaries may not be aware that their provider has a financial interest in recommending IMRT over alternative treatments that may be equally effective, have different risks and side effects, and are less expensive for Medicare and beneficiaries.

ABBREVIATIONS

3D-CRT	three-dimensional conformal radiation therapy
ASTRO	American Society for Radiation Oncology
AUA	American Urological Association
CMS	Centers for Medicare & Medicaid Services
EBRT	external beam radiation therapy
FFS	fee-for-service
HCPCS	Healthcare Common Procedure Coding System
HHS	Department of Health and Human Services
IMRT	intensity-modulated radiation therapy
IOAS	in-office ancillary services
LUGPA	Large Urology Group Practice Association
NPI	national provider identifier
PPACA	Patient Protection and Affordable Care Act
PSA	prostate-specific antigen
SEER	Surveillance Epidemiology and End Results
TIN	taxpayer identification number

* * *

July 19, 2013

Congressional Requesters

Expenditures for Medicare Part B services—which include physician and other outpatient services—have grown rapidly, increasing annually at 5.9 percent, on average, from 2007 through 2011. In comparison, the national economy grew by less than half that rate during the same period. Policymakers have questioned whether some of the growth in spending for Part B services may be attributed to self-referral, which occurs when providers refer their patients to entities—such as themselves or a group practice—in which they or a member of their families have a financial relationship.[1] While federal law generally prohibits self-referral under Medicare, there are exceptions for certain services and arrangements.[2] Among the Medicare diagnostic and therapeutic services that may be self-referred under one of these exceptions is intensity-modulated radiation therapy (IMRT), a form of external beam radiation therapy (EBRT) commonly used to treat prostate cancer. While there are multiple effective treatments for prostate cancer, IMRT is one of the most costly options. In 2010, expenditures for prostate cancer–related IMRT services accounted for about 55 percent of the $1.27 billion that Medicare paid for all IMRT services under Medicare Part B.

Questions have been raised about the effect of self-referral arrangements on the utilization of IMRT services reimbursed under Medicare Part B. Critics of such self-referral arrangements suggest that there may be a financial incentive to overutilize IMRT because diagnosing providers can earn more by self-referring IMRT services than if patients were referred for other treatments.[3] Other treatments for prostate cancer are often considered equally appropriate, as experts have not established a "gold standard" for the treatment of cancer that has not spread beyond the prostate (i.e., localized prostate cancer), which represents a large majority of newly diagnosed prostate cancers.[4] Proponents of self-referral arrangements contend that the self-referral of IMRT services does not affect clinical decision making and that patients benefit from self-referral through, for example, improved coordination among the providers who diagnose and treat patients.

You asked us to examine Medicare self-referral trends among radiation oncology services. In this report, we (1) compare trends in the number of and expenditures for prostate cancer–related IMRT services provided by self-referring and non-self-referring provider groups from 2006 through 2010 and (2) examine how the percentage of prostate cancer patients referred for IMRT may differ on the basis of whether providers self-refer.

To compare trends in the number of and expenditures for prostate cancer–related IMRT services provided by self-referring and non-selfreferring groups in provider offices from 2006 through 2010, we analyzed IMRT delivery claims from the Medicare Part B Carrier file.[5] We identified prostate cancer–related IMRT services using diagnosis codes on the claims. Because there is no indicator or "flag" on the claim that identifies whether services are self-referred or non-self-referred and the Centers for Medicare & Medicaid Services (CMS), the agency that administers Medicare, has no other method for identifying whether a service was self-referred, we developed a claims-based methodology for identifying provider group practices as self-referring or non-self-referring.[6] Specifically, we classified groups as self-referring if the providers who administered IMRT for the group had a financial relationship with the same entity as the provider who referred the IMRT service.[7] Additionally, in order to be considered self-referring, groups had to meet other volume-related criteria, such as self-referring at least half of the courses of IMRT therapy the group provided. To ensure that how we defined our criteria were reliable, we tested alternative thresholds for defining self-referring groups and found that the observed patterns were similar regardless of the threshold used. We also analyzed trends in the utilization of prostate cancer–related IMRT services by whether the service was performed by a limited-specialty or multispecialty group. We defined groups as limited specialty in a given year if more than 75 percent of its office visits were performed by urologists, nonphysician practitioners (e.g., physician assistants), or providers whose specialty was related to the diagnosis or treatment of cancer, such as radiation oncologists. The remaining groups were comprised of providers from a large number of different specialties and were considered multispecialty groups. We examined the trends in prostate–cancer related IMRT services performed in hospital outpatient departments for context.

To examine how the percentage of prostate cancer patients referred for IMRT may differ on the basis of whether providers self-refer, we performed two separate analyses using the Medicare Part B Carrier and hospital outpatient files. First, we compared the percentage of prostate cancer patients that self-referring and non-self-referring providers referred for IMRT and other treatments within a year of being diagnosed in 2007 or 2009. We classified referring providers as self-referring if they were the performing provider on a claim that was paid to a self-referring provider group in the year of, before, or after a beneficiary's prostate cancer diagnosis. All other providers were considered non-self-referring. In addition, we examined how, if at all, the referral patterns for non-selfreferring and self-referring providers were affected by beneficiary characteristics such as age, geographic location (i.e., urban or rural), and beneficiary health.[8] As part of our examination of beneficiary health, we examined how, if at all, provider referral patterns were affected by clinical characteristics of patients' prostate cancers, which were obtained from the New York State Cancer Registry, for beneficiaries who lived in New York and were diagnosed with prostate cancer in either 2007 or 2009. The results of the New York analysis are not generalizable to the entire Medicare population. We used clinical information from the New York State Cancer Registry because such information is not available on Medicare claims, and we determined that the geographic areas included in another common source of such information—Surveillance Epidemiology and End Results (SEER) data—did not sufficiently overlap with areas in which IMRT self-referral was prevalent during our study period. Second, we determined whether the percentage of providers' prostate cancer patients referred for IMRT and other treatments changed after they began to self-refer. Specifically, we identified a group of providers, which we called "switchers," that did not self-refer in 2006 or 2007 but began to self-refer in either 2008 or 2009. We then analyzed the change in the percentage of switchers' newly diagnosed prostate cancer patients referred for IMRT and other treatments before and after switchers began to self-refer. We compared the change for this group of providers to the change among providers who did not begin to self-refer IMRT services during this period. For both analyses, we counted IMRT and other treatments regardless of the setting in which they were performed.

We took several steps to ensure that the data used to produce this report were sufficiently reliable. Specifically, we assessed the reliability of the CMS data we used by interviewing officials responsible for overseeing these data sources, reviewing relevant documentation, and examining the data for obvious errors. We determined that the data were sufficiently reliable for the purposes of our study. (See app. I for more details on our scope and methodology.)

We conducted this performance audit from May 2010 through July 2013 in accordance with generally accepted government auditing standards. Those standards require that we plan and perform the audit to obtain sufficient, appropriate evidence to provide a reasonable basis for our findings and conclusions based on our audit objectives. We believe that the evidence obtained provides a reasonable basis for our findings and conclusions based on our audit objectives.

BACKGROUND

Prostate cancer patients choose among multiple treatments that are often considered equally appropriate but can have different risks and side effects. The treatments can also vary in cost, with IMRT being one of the most costly options.

Diagnosis and Treatment of Prostate Cancer

Cancer of the prostate—a gland located at the base of the urinary bladder—is the second most common cancer among men in the United States, with approximately 1 in 6 men receiving a diagnosis of prostate cancer in his lifetime.[9] In 2010, there were an estimated 218,000 new cases of prostate cancer and approximately 32,000 deaths due to prostate cancer. Most men in the United States are diagnosed with prostate cancer as a result of an abnormal digital rectal exam or prostate-specific antigen test. After an abnormal test result, beneficiaries often undergo a prostate biopsy, during which a provider—typically a urologist—removes small amounts of prostate tissue. Another provider then examines the tissue to determine whether a beneficiary has prostate cancer.

IMRT is one of multiple treatment options available to patients with prostate cancer. The type of treatment a prostate cancer patient chooses depends on a number of different factors such as life expectancy, overall health, personal preferences, provider recommendations, and the clinical characteristics of a patient's prostate cancer. For many men, multiple treatment options are considered equally appropriate.[10] For instance, IMRT, brachytherapy, and a radical prostatectomy are all among the treatments considered appropriate for men with low-risk prostate cancer.[11]

Even though such treatments are often considered equally appropriate, the risks and side effects for each treatment are different. Compared to IMRT, prostate cancer patients undergoing a radical prostatectomy have a higher rate of short term urinary problems and erectile dysfunction but do not face bowel-related side effects, which are experienced by some men undergoing IMRT.[12]

Compared to IMRT, prostate cancer patients undergoing brachytherapy have lower rates of bowel-related side effects but about 1 in 10 patients undergoing brachytherapy experience acute urinary retention.

Also, several studies have reported that physician recommendations play a large role in influencing a patient's decision,[13] and another study found that the use of a particular prostate cancer treatment decreased after its payment was reduced, suggesting that financial incentives may have influenced treatment decisions.[14]

Currently, providers who self-refer IMRT services are generally not required to disclose to their patients that they have a financial interest in the service.[15] Some common prostate cancer treatments are summarized in table 1.

Table 1. Prostate Cancer Treatments

Treatment	Description
Radical prostatectomy	A radical prostatectomy is a surgical procedure in which the entire prostate gland is removed. A prostatectomy can be performed with or without robotic assistance.
Three-dimensional conformal radiation therapy (3D-CRT)	3D-CRT is a form of external beam radiation therapy (EBRT) during which multiple doses of radiation from an external source are administered over several weeks. In 3D-CRT, radiation beams are shaped in an attempt to maximize the amount of radiation the tumor receives and reduce the amount of radiation to which normal tissue is exposed.
Intensity-modulated radiation therapy (IMRT)	IMRT is a newer and an even more precise form of EBRT that allows even more radiation to be delivered to the tumor while sparing normal tissue.
Brachytherapy	Brachytherapy is a treatment that involves the implantation of radioactive sources directly inside the prostate.
Active surveillance	Active surveillance is a regimen of following a patient's condition without giving any treatment, unless the patient's condition changes. An exact regimen has not been established for active surveillance. However, typical protocols involve periodic physical examination, prostate-specific antigen testing, and repeat prostate biopsies.
Hormone therapy	Hormone therapy is a treatment that removes or blocks the actions of male sex hormones, which can cause prostate cancer to grow, in order to stop the growth of prostate cancer. Drugs, surgery, or other hormones are used to reduce hormone production or block their effects.
Other treatments	Other treatments for prostate cancer include stereotactic body radiotherapy / stereotactic radiosurgery (forms of EBRT during which beneficiaries receive larger daily doses of radiation over a shorter period of time), cryosurgery (freezing prostate cancer by injecting gases through thin needles inserted into the prostate), and proton beam therapy (a form ofEBRT that involves the use of particles—protons—rather than photons, which are used in the majority of EBRT treatments).

Source: GAO analysis of published literature.

Medicare Reimbursement for IMRT Services and Costs of Treatment Options for Prostate Cancer

Medicare reimbursement rates for IMRT delivery services varied over time, and rates are not directly comparable between settings. Beneficiaries receive approximately 45 separate IMRT delivery services over several weeks during a course of IMRT to treat prostate cancer. Medicare beneficiaries predominantly receive IMRT delivery services in two settings—physician offices or hospital outpatient departments. The Medicare reimbursement per IMRT delivery service increased from approximately $319 to $421 from 2006 to 2010 and then to $484 by 2013 for services performed in hospital outpatient departments.[16] For services performed in physician offices, the reimbursement rate decreased from approximately $690 to $511 from 2006 to 2010 and then to $406 by 2013.[17] The reimbursement rates for IMRT delivery services performed in physician offices and hospital outpatient departments are not directly comparable. For instance, if an IMRT delivery service was performed in a hospital outpatient department, payment includes the technical component for image guidance,[18] which is almost always furnished with an IMRT service. In physician offices, image guidance is reimbursed separately.

Researchers have consistently found that courses of IMRT, which include IMRT delivery and other services,[19] are more costly than other treatments for prostate cancer, with the exception of proton therapy.[20] Researchers have found IMRT to be more costly despite differences among studies in design and methodology, such as the services counted toward total treatment costs, the duration of time during which costs are studied (e.g., first year costs vs. lifetime costs), and the patient population studied. One recent study found that, among men diagnosed with prostate cancer in 2005, the cost to Medicare per course of treatment was approximately $14,000 to $15,000 higher for men receiving IMRT ($31,574) than for men who received brachytherapy ($17,076) or a prostatectomy ($16,469 or $16,762, depending on the type of prostatectomy).[21] Despite the 2013 reduction in the Medicare reimbursement rate for IMRT delivery services performed in physician offices, we found that IMRT remains substantially more expensive than other treatments for prostate cancer, with the exception of proton therapy.[22]

NUMBER OF AND EXPENDITURES FOR PROSTATE CANCER–RELATED IMRT SERVICES PROVIDED BY SELF-REFERRING GROUPS GREW RAPIDLY, WHILE DECLINING FOR NON-SELF-REFERRING GROUPS

We found that the number of and expenditures for Medicare prostate cancer–related IMRT services performed by self-referring groups grew rapidly from 2006 through 2010. In contrast, the number of and Medicare expenditures for prostate cancer–related IMRT services performed by non-self-referring groups declined over the period.

Number of Prostate Cancer–Related IMRT Services Performed Increased among Self-Referring Groups— Specifically, Limited-Specialty Groups— and Decreased among NonSelf-Referring Groups

From 2006 through 2010, the number of prostate cancer–related IMRT services performed by self-referring groups increased rapidly, while the number performed by non-self-referring groups decreased. The number of prostate cancer–related IMRT services performed by self-referring groups increased from approximately 80,000 to 366,000, an annual growth rate of 46 percent (see figure 1). Consistent with that growth, the number of self-referring groups also increased rapidly over the period. In contrast, the number of prostate cancer–related IMRT services performed by non-self-referring groups in physician offices decreased from approximately 490,000 to 466,000, an annual decrease of 1 percent.

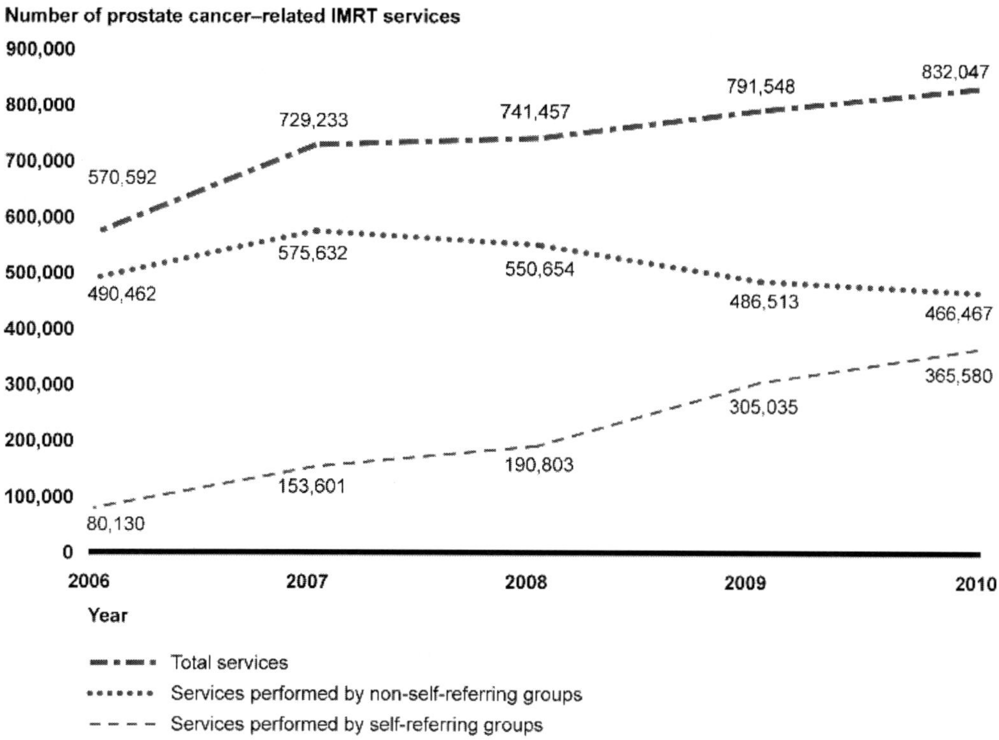

Source: GAO analysis of CMS data.

Figure 1. Number of Medicare Prostate Cancer–Related IMRT Services Performed by Self-Referring and Non-Self-Referring Groups in Physician Offices, 2006-2010.

The rapid increase in prostate cancer–related IMRT services performed by self-referring groups coincided with several other trends from 2006 through 2010. First, the number of prostate-cancer related IMRT services performed in hospital outpatient departments and by self-referring and non-self-referring groups all grew from 2006 to 2007. After 2007, the rapid increase in prostate cancer–related IMRT services performed by self-referring groups coincided with declines in these services within hospital outpatient departments and among non-self-referring groups. Overall utilization of prostate cancer–related IMRT services therefore remained relatively flat across these settings after 2007, indicating a shift away from hospital outpatient departments and non-self-referring groups and toward self-referring groups. (See app. II for information on the trends in IMRT services performed in hospital outpatient departments.) Second, while the number of prostate cancer–related IMRT services provided to Medicare fee-for-service (FFS) beneficiaries has stabilized since 2007, the percentage of newly diagnosed Medicare beneficiaries receiving IMRT has increased.[23] While seemingly contradictory, these two trends occurring simultaneously can in part be explained by (1) a decrease in the total number of Medicare FFS beneficiaries from 2006 through 2010[24] and (2) a decrease in the number of men newly diagnosed with prostate cancer.[25] Third, the increasing percentage of prostate cancer patients receiving IMRT may partially be explained by a shift from an older form of EBRT—3D-CRT—to a newer form—IMRT, though the largest effect of this substitution likely occurred earlier in our study period as IMRT largely replaced 3D-CRT by 2007.[26]

Our analysis showed that, from 2006 through 2010, the growth in prostate cancer–related IMRT services performed by self-referring groups was entirely due to an increase in the services performed by limited-specialty groups (see figure 2). Limited-specialty groups were comprised of urologists and a small number of other specialties.[27] Over our study period, the number of prostate cancer–related IMRT services performed by limited-specialty self-referring groups increased over fivefold, from approximately 56,000 to 343,000. In contrast, the number of such services performed by multispecialty self-referring groups, which were comprised of a large number of different provider types, declined slightly, going from approximately 23,000 to 22,000.

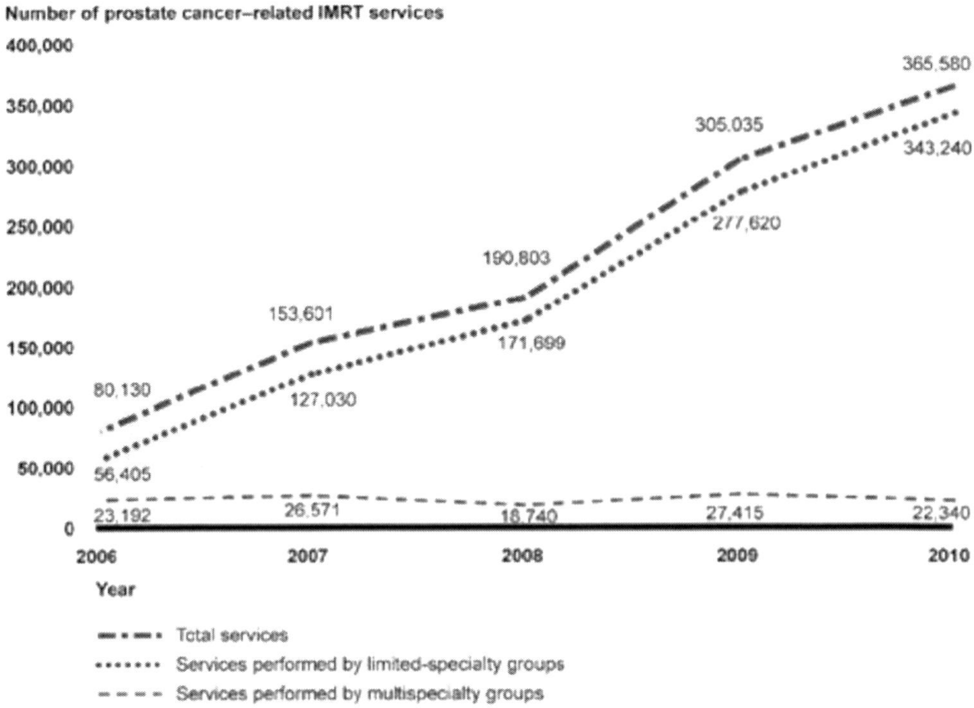

Source: GAO analysis of CMS data.

Notes: In 2006 and 2008, less than 1 percent of total services could not be attributed to either limited-specialty or multispecialty groups. We defined groups as limited specialty in a given year if more than 75 percent of its office visits were performed by urologists, nonphysician practitioners (e.g., physician assistants), or providers whose specialty was related to the diagnosis or treatment of cancer, such as radiation oncologists. The remaining groups were comprised of providers from a large number of different specialties and were considered multispecialty groups.

Figure 2. Number of Medicare Prostate Cancer–Related IMRT Services Performed by Limited-Specialty and Multispecialty Self-Referring Groups, 2006-2010.

Expenditures for Prostate Cancer–Related IMRT Services Performed by Self-Referring Groups Increased Rapidly, while Declining for Non-Self-Referring Groups

Medicare expenditures for prostate cancer–related IMRT services performed by self-referring groups increased rapidly from 2006 through 2010, while decreasing for services performed by non-self-referring groups. Specifically, expenditures for prostate cancer–related IMRT services performed by self-referring groups increased from $52 million to $190 million, an average increase of 38 percent a year (see figure 3). In contrast, expenditures for prostate cancer–related IMRT services performed by non-self-referring groups in physician offices declined by an average of 8 percent a year. For comparison, expenditures for prostate cancer–related IMRT services performed in hospital outpatient departments grew an average of 7 percent a year during the period we studied. (For more information about hospital outpatient department expenditure trends, see app. II.)

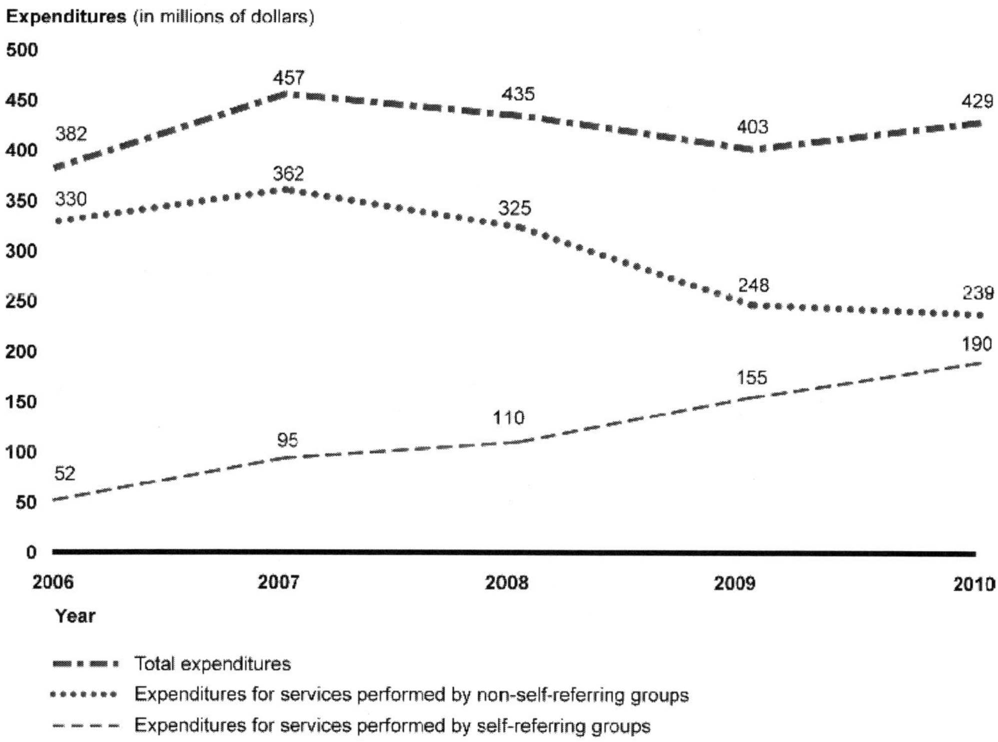

Source: GAO analysis of CMS data.

Figure 3. Changes in Medicare Prostate Cancer–Related IMRT Expenditures for Services Performed by Self-Referring and Non-Self-Referring Provider Groups in Physician Offices, 2006-2010.

Self-Referring Providers Referred Their Prostate Cancer Patients for IMRT More Frequently than Non-Self-Referring Providers

Self-referring providers were more likely to refer their Medicare prostate cancer patients for IMRT and less likely to refer them for other treatments when compared to non-self-referring providers. In addition, after providers began self-referring IMRT services, they substantially increased the percentage of their prostate cancer patients they referred for IMRT, in contrast to providers who did not begin to self-refer IMRT services during the same period.

Self-Referring Providers Were 53 Percent More Likely to Refer Their Prostate Cancer Patients for IMRT than Non-SelfReferring Providers

Self-referring providers were more likely to refer their prostate cancer patients for IMRT and less likely to refer them for other treatments compared to non-self-referring providers. Self-referring providers referred approximately 52 percent of their patients who were newly diagnosed with prostate cancer in 2009 for IMRT, while non-self-referring providers referred 34 percent of their patients for IMRT (see table 2). Self-referring providers also referred a lower percentage of their prostate cancer patients for nearly all other types of treatments compared to non-selfreferring providers, with the largest differences among patients being referred for brachytherapy or a radical prostatectomy.[28] Other differences were smaller—self-referring providers were about 8 percent less likely to refer their patients for active surveillance compared to non-self-referring providers. (For alternative groupings in which beneficiaries are sorted into discrete treatment categories, see app. III.)

The difference between self-referring and non-self-referring providers in the percentage of their prostate cancer patients referred for IMRT was largely due to self-referring providers who belonged to limited-specialty groups. Self-referring providers who belonged to a limited-specialty group referred approximately 52 percent of their patients diagnosed with prostate cancer in 2007 or 2009 for IMRT.[29] In contrast, self-referring providers who belonged to a multispecialty group referred approximately 36 percent of their patients diagnosed with prostate cancer in 2007 or 2009 for IMRT, only moderately higher than the 33 percent of non-selfreferring providers' patients diagnosed with prostate cancer in 2007 or 2009 who were referred for IMRT.

Differences in the percentage of prostate cancer patients referred for IMRT between self-referring and non-self-referring providers persisted after accounting for differences in age, geographic location (i.e., urban or rural), and beneficiary health, including clinical characteristics of prostate cancers for a subset of beneficiaries who lived in New York.

Table 2. Percentage of Self-Referring and Non-Self-Referring Providers' Medicare Patients Referred for a Given Treatment after a Diagnosis of Prostate Cancer in 2009

Prostate cancer treatment	Percentage of non-self-referring providers' patients referred for a given treatment (N=48,298)	Percentage of self-referring providers' patients referred for a given treatment (N=9,991)	Percentage point difference	Percentage more or less likely self-referring providers were torefer patients for a given treatment compared to non-self-referring providers
Intensity-modulated radiation therapy	33.7%	51.7%	18.0	53.5%
Active surveillance	22.9	21.0	-1.9	-8.2
Radical prostatectomy	18.0	13.1	-4.9	-27.0
Hormone therapy only[a]	11.4	7.7	-3.8	-32.9
Brachytherapy	14.0	7.0	-7.0	-50.0
Other treatments[b]	6.0	3.2	-2.8	-46.5
Three-dimensional conformal radiation therapy / other external beam radiation therapy	2.4	1.1	-1.3	-55.2

Source: GAO analysis of CMS data.

Notes: Treatment categories do not sum to 100 percent because, with the exception of active surveillance and hormone therapy only, a patient was counted in more than one treatment category if he received a combination of therapies. Including combinations involving hormone therapy, self-referring and non-self-referring providers referred nearly equal percentages of their patients for a combination of treatments—27 percent and 26 percent, respectively.

[a]Prostate cancer patients also commonly receive hormone therapy in conjunction with other treatments. Self-referring providers referred 31.9 percent of their prostate cancer patients for any hormone therapy, while non-self-referring providers referred 33.7 percent.

[b]"Other treatments" consists of cryoablation, stereotactic body radiotherapy / stereotactic radiosurgery, and proton therapy. Self-referring providers were less likely to refer their patients for cryoablation and stereotactic body radiotherapy / stereotactic radiosurgery compared to non-selfreferring providers, but both types of providers referred the same percentage of their patients for proton therapy—approximately 1 percent.

Age

Differences between self-referring and non-self-referring providers in the percentage of prostate cancer patients that were referred for IMRT could not be explained by differences in age. The average age when a beneficiary was diagnosed with prostate cancer was the same for patients of both self-referring and non-self-referring providers, and, regardless of their patients' ages, self-referring providers were more likely to refer their patients for IMRT compared to non-self-referring providers. The average age when a beneficiary was diagnosed with prostate cancer was 74 years old for patients of both self-referring and non-self-referring providers. Depending on the age range, self-referring providers were anywhere from 48 percent to 62 percent more likely to refer their patients for IMRT compared to non-self-referring providers. For more information about how the percentage of prostate cancer patients referred for IMRT and other treatments by self-referring and non-self-referring providers changed on the basis of the age of a beneficiary, see appendix IV.

Geographic Location

Differences between self-referring and non-self-referring providers in the percentage of prostate cancer patients that were referred for IMRT could not be explained by differences in geographic location. Self-referring providers were more likely to refer their patients for IMRT compared to non-self-referring providers, regardless of differences in geographic location.[30] Self-referring providers were 52 percent more likely to refer their patients that lived in urban areas for IMRT compared to non-selfreferring providers. Similarly, self-referring providers were 42 percent more likely to refer their patients that lived in rural areas for IMRT compared to non-self-referring providers.

Beneficiary Health

Differences between self-referring and non-self-referring providers in the percentage of prostate cancer patients that were referred for IMRT could not be explained by differences in beneficiary health. Self-referring and non-self-referring providers' prostate cancer patients had a similar average health status, and self-referring providers were more likely to refer their patients for IMRT compared to non-self-referring providers, regardless of whether their patients had low-, intermediate-, or high-risk prostate cancer. Self-referring providers' patients had an average risk score—a proxy for health status—of 0.94 in 2009, and non-self-referring providers' patients had an average risk score of 0.92, indicating that the two patient populations had a similar average health status.[31] In cases where we had information on the clinical characteristics of patients' prostate cancer, we found that self-referring providers were more likely than non-self-referring providers to refer their patients for IMRT, although the difference decreased as prostate cancer risk level increased. Specifically, self-referring providers were 91 percent, 41 percent, and 33 percent more likely than non-self-referring providers to refer patients with low-, intermediate-, and high-risk prostate cancer for IMRT, respectively.[32] The difference in IMRT referrals made by self-referring and non-self-referring providers narrowed as patients' prostate cancer risk level increased in part because non-self-referring providers increased IMRT referrals and decreased brachytherapy referrals as cancer risk levels increased. In comparison, self-referring providers referred similarly small percentages of patients for brachytherapy for all three risk levels, and their IMRT referrals increased only moderately as their patients' risk level increased.[33]

Providers Substantially Increased the Percentage of Their Prostate Cancer Patients They Referred for IMRT after They Began to Self-Refer

Providers that switched from being non-self-referring to self-referring— that is, switchers—referred a greater percentage of their prostate cancer patients for IMRT after they began to self-refer (see table 3). Specifically, switchers referred 37 percent of their patients who were diagnosed with prostate cancer in 2007 for IMRT. After beginning to self-refer, switchers referred 54 percent of their patients who were diagnosed with prostate cancer in

2009 for IMRT. While providers that did not begin to self-refer— that is, self-referrers and non-self-referrers—referred different percentages of their patients who were diagnosed with prostate cancer in 2007 for IMRT, the percentages of their patients they referred for IMRT remained relatively consistent over the same period when switchers dramatically increased the percentage of their patients they referred for IMRT. This suggests that the increase seen among switchers was likely not due to provider characteristics that were relatively stable over time or changes in the way all providers treated prostate cancer in response to such things as changing treatment guidelines. (See app. V for more information about how the percentage of beneficiaries switchers, non-selfreferring providers, and self-referring providers referred for a given treatment.)

Table 3. Change in the Percentage of Medicare Prostate Cancer Patients Providers Referred for IMRT after a Diagnosis of Prostate Cancer in 2007 or 2009

Type of provider	Percentage of providers' patients referred for IMRT among beneficiaries diagnosed in 2007	Percentage of providers' patients referred for IMRT among beneficiaries diagnosed in 2009	Percentage point change from 2007 to 2009	Percentage more or lesslikely providers were torefer patients for IMRT in 2009 compared to 2007
Non-self-referring	31.4%	33.1%	1.7	5.5%
Self-referring	55.7	52.9	-2.8	-5.1
Switcher	37.0	54.2	17.2	46.6

Source: GAO analysis of CMS data.

Notes: We define switchers as those providers that did not self-refer in 2006 or 2007 but began to self-refer in either 2008 or 2009. In 2007, switchers, self-referring providers, and non-self-referring providers referred 4,903, 1,776, and 42,471 prostate cancer patients for treatment, respectively. In 2009, switchers, self-referring providers, and non-self-referring providers referred 4,156, 1,244, and 34,107 prostate cancer patients for treatment, respectively.

CONCLUSION

IMRT has been shown to be an effective treatment option for localized prostate cancer and allows radiation to be delivered to the tumor while minimizing damage to normal tissue. Proponents of self-referral arrangements contend that the self-referral of IMRT services does not affect clinical decision making and that patients benefit from self-referral through, for example, improved coordination among the providers who diagnose and treat patients. However, our review indicates that Medicare providers that self-referred IMRT services—particularly those practicing in limited-specialty groups—were substantially more likely to refer their prostate cancer patients for IMRT and less likely to refer them for other, less costly treatments, especially brachytherapy or a radical prostatectomy, compared to providers who did not self-refer. The relatively higher rate of IMRT referrals among self-referring providers cannot be explained by beneficiary age, geographic location, or health. Consistent with these findings, we also found that after providers began to self-refer IMRT services they substantially increased the percentage of their prostate cancer patients they referred for IMRT, while providers that did not begin to self-refer experienced much smaller changes over the same period. Taken together, our findings suggest that financial incentives were likely a major factor driving the increase of IMRT referrals among self-referring providers in limited-specialty groups.

The greater use of IMRT by self-referring Medicare providers to treat prostate cancer raises two potential concerns. First, because physician recommendations play a large role in influencing a patient's treatment decision, a financial interest in one treatment option may diminish the role that other criteria—such as life expectancy, overall health, patient preferences, and clinical characteristics of the prostate cancer—play in the decision-making process. Despite the fact that several treatment options are often considered equally appropriate, the higher use of IMRT among providers who self-refer seems problematic because prostate cancer treatments differ in terms of their risks and side effects, such as the likelihood of developing sexual, urinary, or bowel-related side effects. To the extent that providers' financial interests are shaping treatment decisions, some patients may end up on a treatment course that does not best meet their individual needs. Second, because IMRT costs more than most other treatments, the higher use of IMRT by self-referring providers results in higher costs for Medicare and beneficiaries. To the extent that treatment decisions are driven by providers' financial interest and not by patient preference, these increased costs are difficult to justify.

Given self-referral's potential effect on both the Medicare program and beneficiaries, it is imperative that CMS improve its ability to identify and monitor the effects of such services. CMS is not currently well-positioned to address self-referring providers' financial incentive to refer their prostate cancer patients for IMRT, as CMS currently does not have a method for easily identifying such services. Without a way to identify self-referred services, such as a self-referral flag on Medicare Part B claims, CMS does not have the ongoing ability to monitor self-referral and its effects on beneficiary treatment selection and costs to both Medicare and beneficiaries.

In addition, Medicare providers who self-refer IMRT services are generally not required to disclose their financial interest in IMRT. Thus, beneficiaries may not be aware that their provider has an incentive to recommend IMRT over alternative treatments which may be equally effective, have different risks and side effects, and are less expensive for Medicare and beneficiaries. Beneficiaries need to select among different prostate cancer treatment options, and beneficiary knowledge of a referring provider's financial interest in IMRT may be an important consideration in making these selections. Currently, the Department of Health and Human Services (HHS), the agency that administers CMS, lacks the authority to establish a disclosure protocol for providers who self-refer IMRT services.

Matter for Congressional Consideration

To increase beneficiaries' awareness of providers' financial interest in a particular treatment, Congress should consider directing the Secretary of Health and Human Services to require providers who self-refer IMRT services to disclose to their patients that they have a financial interest in the service.

Recommendation for Executive Action

We recommend that the Administrator of CMS insert a self-referral flag on its Medicare Part B claims form, require providers to indicate whether the IMRT service for which a provider bills Medicare is self-referred, and monitor the effects that self-referral has on costs and beneficiary treatment selection.

Agency and Third-Party Comments and Our Evaluation

We provided a draft of this report to HHS for comment. HHS provided. We also obtained oral comments from representatives of three professional associations selected because they represent stakeholders with specific involvement in prostate cancer–related IMRT services.

The three associations were the American Society for Radiation Oncology (ASTRO), which represents radiation oncologists; the American Urological Association (AUA), which represents urologists; and the Large Urology Group Practice Association (LUGPA), which represents large urology group practices. We summarize and respond to comments from HHS and representatives from the three professional associations in the following sections.

HHS Comments

In its comments, HHS stated that it did not concur with our recommendation. HHS did not comment on the matter for congressional consideration or the main finding of the report—that self-referring providers, particularly those belonging to limited-specialty groups, referred a substantially higher percentage of their prostate cancer patients for IMRT.

HHS did not concur with our recommendation that CMS insert a self-referral flag on its Medicare Part B claims form, require providers to indicate whether the IMRT service for which a provider bills Medicare is self-referred, and monitor the effects that self-referral has on costs and beneficiary treatment selection. HHS stated that flagging self-referred services and tracking their effects would not address overutilization that occurs as a result of self-referral, would be complex to administer, and may have unintended consequences, which HHS did not delineate. In addition, HHS stated that the President's fiscal year 2014 budget proposal includes a provision to exclude certain services from the in-office ancillary services (IOAS) exception. To the extent that self-referral for IMRT services continues to be permitted, we believe that including an indicator or flag on the claims would be an effective way to identify and track self-referral and would give CMS the ability to analyze the effects of self-referral on utilization patterns. Furthermore, we do not believe an indicator or flag on the claims would be complex to administer, as CMS requires providers to use similar indicators to provide additional information about certain other services.

On the basis of HHS's written response to our report, we are concerned that HHS does not appear to recognize the effects IMRT self-referral can have on beneficiaries and the Medicare program. HHS did not comment on our matter for congressional consideration or our key finding that self-referring providers, particularly those belonging to limited specialty groups, referred a substantially higher percentage of their prostate cancer patients for IMRT.

Given the magnitude of these findings, we continue to believe that CMS should take steps to monitor the impact that IMRT self-referral has on costs and treatment selection.

HHS also provided technical comments that we incorporated as appropriate.

Professional Association Comments

American Society for Radiation Oncology

ASTRO representatives generally agreed with our findings but thought our recommendation and matter for congressional consideration should be stronger. They said we should recommend that Congress close the IOAS exception because the findings from the report, in combination with previous self-referral research we and others have published, indicate the necessity for such an action. An examination of the IOAS was beyond the scope of our work. To the extent that IMRT self-referral is still permissible, ASTRO representatives also said that inserting a self-referral flag would not be an effective way to identify self-referral. Instead, they suggested implementing reporting requirements similar to the financial transparency requirements for physician-owned specialty hospitals under PPACA and requiring self-referring providers to indicate on their Medicare provider enrollment forms their financial interest in referrals. Further, ASTRO representatives said that self-referring providers should be required to notify patients that they may receive IMRT at alternative locations and that other treatment options are available. We continue to believe that inserting a self-referral flag on Medicare Part B claims would be an effective way to track and monitor self-referral and that beneficiary awareness of their providers' financial interests is important. However, to the extent that other strategies exist that would allow CMS to increase beneficiary awareness and monitor self-referral, such efforts would be consistent with the intent of our recommendation and matter for congressional consideration.

American Urological Association

AUA representatives said we did not have sufficient evidence to link financial incentives to the increase in IMRT use among self-referring providers and disagreed with our conclusion that financial incentives for self-referring providers belonging to limited specialty groups were likely a major factor driving the increase in the percentage of prostate cancer patients referred for IMRT. Specifically, AUA representatives said the flat trend in the utilization of prostate cancer-related IMRT services from 2007 through 2010 indicates utilization has simply shifted from hospital outpatient departments to physician offices and that this trend undermines our conclusion that financial incentives increase IMRT use. As explained in our report, the trend in the percentage of patients newly diagnosed with prostate cancer referred for IMRT was not flat; instead, it increased over the study period. This increase occurred while the utilization of IMRT services remained about the same in part because the annual number of Medicare FFS beneficiaries who were diagnosed with prostate cancer declined by about 20 percent over our study period. In addition, we found that self-referring providers, which were predominantly from limited-specialty groups, referred a higher percentage of their Medicare FFS patients for IMRT than did other providers and that their higher IMRT referral rate could not be explained by differences in age, geographic location, or beneficiary health. As a result, we continue to believe that financial incentives were likely a major factor driving the higher IMRT referral rate of self-referring providers from limited-specialty groups.

AUA representatives had several other critiques of our report. Specifically, they indicated that we did not put enough emphasis on the patient's role in choosing a treatment and expressed concern that we did not include more clinical information on patients' prostate cancer, such as information on cancer stage and grade, or include Medicare Advantage beneficiaries in our study population. We address two of these critiques in the report. Specifically, we note that patient preference is one of many factors that affect a beneficiary's treatment decision, and we include clinical information on patients' prostate cancer for a subset of beneficiaries from New York.[34] However, we did not include Medicare Advantage beneficiaries in our study population because Medicare Advantage plans are not required to submit claims to CMS, and, thus, we do not have detailed information on the services Medicare Advantage beneficiaries receive or the providers who refer and perform those services.

Finally, AUA representatives stated that the declining percentage of self-referring providers' patients referred for brachytherapy from 2007 to 2009 could reflect a change in practice standards, as they said brachytherapy is no longer recommended as a sole treatment for intermediate- and high-risk prostate cancer. While we note that brachytherapy use has declined even among providers who do not self-refer, we do not believe that changing guidelines or the possibility of differences in guideline adherence between non-self-referring and self-referring providers could explain in totality why self-referring providers refer a smaller percentage of their patients for brachytherapy. First, self-referring providers referred a substantially lower percentage of their patients for brachytherapy, even after accounting for the decline in brachytherapy use for both non-selfreferring and self-referring providers from 2007 to 2009. Second, among those patients for whom we had clinical data, the biggest differences in IMRT and brachytherapy use between self-referring and non-self-referring providers were for patients with low-risk cancer, which would not be affected by the change in practice guidelines for intermediate- and high-risk prostate cancer the AUA representatives referenced.

Large Urology Group Practice Association

LUGPA representatives disagreed with our conclusion that financial incentives for self-referring providers—specifically those in limited-specialty groups—were likely a major factor driving the increase in the percentage of prostate cancer patients referred for IMRT. Instead, they said patient preference and an increase in the number of self-referring providers explain the increase in IMRT utilization by self-referring providers. While we did not perform our trend analysis at the provider level, we do note in the report that the number of self-referring groups increased substantially over our study period. This corresponds with a shift in the location where patients received IMRT, from hospital outpatient departments to physician offices. However, these trends that we note do not negate our analysis of the referral patterns of self-referring providers. Specifically, self-referring providers who belonged to a limited-specialty group referred a higher percentage of their newly diagnosed prostate cancer patients for IMRT, and, thus, the increased number of self-referring providers has also resulted in a higher percentage of patients receiving IMRT. Also, LUPGA representatives said the increase in the percentage of self-referring providers' patients referred for IMRT could be due to such patients more frequently consulting with radiation oncologists before initiating treatment, which one study indicated leads to higher utilization of radiation therapy, defined as EBRT or brachytherapy.[35] We believe it is unlikely that access to a radiation oncologist drove the differences in IMRT referrals between self-referring and non-self-referring providers because self-referring providers who belonged to a multispecialty group referred a substantially lower percentage of their patients for IMRT compared to self-referring providers who belonged to a limited-specialty group, despite the likelihood that patients in both instances had access to a radiation oncologist within the group practice.

LUGPA raised several other points of concern about our review. First, LUGPA representatives said our assertion that IMRT, brachytherapy, and a prostatectomy are clinically equivalent treatments is inappropriate. We disagree with LUGPA's characterization of our discussion of IMRT, brachytherapy, and a prostatectomy as treatment options. We recognize that these treatments are not equally appropriate for all men diagnosed with prostate cancer and do not assert that in our report. Rather, we say that these treatments are often—not always—considered equally appropriate and give an example of when they are considered equally appropriate—men with low-risk prostate cancer. We also recognize that, for any particular patient, a given treatment might not be appropriate due to considerations such as age and comorbidities. Second, LUGPA representatives said that we did not acknowledge that all sites of services have essentially identical financial incentives to perform services for which they receive compensation. They said our work showed the percentage of newly diagnosed prostate cancer patients referred for active surveillance was nearly equal between self-referring and non-selfreferring providers and that this was evidence that self-referring providers treat patients based on patient choice and sound clinical decision making. We disagree with LUGPA's assertion that the percentage of newly diagnosed prostate cancer patients referred for active surveillance was nearly equal between self-referring and non-self-referring providers, as self-referring providers were approximately 8 percent less likely to refer their patients for active surveillance than were non-self-referring providers. As we note in the report, IMRT is more costly than other treatments for prostate cancer, resulting in a financial incentive for self-referring providers to refer their patients for IMRT over other treatments. We found that self-referring providers referred a higher percentage of their patients for IMRT than did non-self-referring providers and that the difference in IMRT referral rates could not be explained by variations in patient age, geographic location, or patient health status. As a result, we continue to believe that self-referring providers' higher IMRT referral rates are driven by a financial incentive for these providers to refer newly diagnosed prostate cancer patients for IMRT. Third, LUGPA representatives said we should have studied the use of IMRT for conditions other than prostate cancer. The use of IMRT to treat other conditions was outside the scope of our work. Finally, LUGPA representatives indicated that our estimates of 3D-CRT utilization for newly diagnosed prostate cancer patients are too low. We believe our calculation of the percentage of patients who were newly diagnosed with prostate cancer in 2009 and referred for 3D-CRT is accurate. We solicited input from multiple physician associations, including members of LUGPA, regarding the appropriate HCPCS codes to use to track 3D-CRT and examined 100 percent of claims from the Medicare Carrier and hospital outpatient department files to identify all 3D-CRT services received by newly diagnosed prostate cancer patients.

James C. Cosgrove
Director, Health Care

APPENDIX I: SCOPE AND METHODS

This section describes the scope and methodology used to analyze our two objectives: (1) comparing trends in the number of and expenditures for Medicare prostate cancer–related intensity-modulated radiation therapy (IMRT) services provided by self-referring and non-self-referring groups from 2006 through 2010 and (2) examining how the percentage of Medicare prostate cancer patients referred for IMRT may differ on the basis of whether providers self-refer.

To compare trends in the number of and expenditures for prostate cancer–related IMRT services provided in physician offices or hospital outpatient departments from 2006 through 2010, we analyzed IMRT claims from the Medicare Part B Carrier and hospital outpatient files.[1] We identified IMRT services on the basis of Healthcare Common Procedure Coding System (HCPCS) codes associated with the delivery of IMRT— 77418 and 0073T.[2] We classified IMRT services as related to prostate cancer if the principal diagnosis code was 185 or 233.4—malignant neoplasm of the prostate or carcinoma in situ of prostate, respectively—or if one of these codes was billed on an IMRT claim and no other diagnosis code related to another cancer was billed on the same claim.

To determine whether prostate cancer–related IMRT services from 2006 through 2010 were performed by self-referring or non-self-referring provider groups, we first limited our analysis to only those IMRT services in the Medicare Part B Carrier file. [3] Because there is no indicator or "flag" on the claim that identifies whether services are self-referred or non-self-referred and the Centers for Medicare & Medicaid Services (CMS), the agency that administers Medicare, has no other method for identifying whether a service was self-referred, we developed a claims-based methodology for identifying provider group practices as self-referring or non-self-referring.[4] We classified groups, identified by taxpayer identification numbers (TIN)—an identification number used by the Internal Revenue Service—as self-referring in a given year if: (1) we could identify a prostate biopsy for at least 50 percent of the prostate cancer–related IMRT episodes provided by groups,[5] (2) at least 50 percent of these episodes were self-referred, and (3) a group had a minimum number of 10 self-referred IMRT episodes.[6] The remaining groups were considered non-self-referring.[7] To ensure that how we defined our criteria were reliable, we tested alternative thresholds for defining self-referring groups and found that, regardless of specification, the rapid growth of services performed by self-referring groups persisted and that the growth was due to limited-specialty groups. A patient's episode of prostate cancer–related IMRT was considered self-referred if the provider who performed his prostate biopsy and the performing provider(s) on the IMRT claim(s) billed to the same TIN in the year(s) the IMRT services were performed, the year the biopsy was performed, or the year between, if applicable.[8] To find prostate biopsies for beneficiaries, we searched through 2 years of their claims history to find the prostate biopsy nearest to, but not after, the date of their first IMRT service. If a beneficiary received multiple episodes of IMRT from 2006 through 2010, we searched back 2 years from the date of the first IMRT service for each episode. We further defined self-referring provider groups as either limited-specialty or multispecialty groups. We defined groups as limited specialty if more than 75 percent of its office visits in a given year were performed by urologists, nonphysician practitioners, or physicians whose specialty was related to the diagnosis or treatment of cancer, such as radiation oncologists. The remaining self-referring groups were comprised of providers from a large number of different specialties and were considered multispecialty groups.

To examine how the percentage of prostate cancer patients referred for IMRT may differ on the basis of whether providers self-refer, we first identified a list of Medicare beneficiaries who were newly diagnosed with prostate cancer in 2007 or 2009. We used a Medicare claims-derived date from the Chronic Condition Data Warehouse (CCDW), a CMS database, that indicates the first occurrence of prostate cancer as a proxy for the date on which a beneficiary was diagnosed with prostate cancer. We further narrowed the list of prostate cancer patients we studied to those who (1) were at least 66 years of age on their date of diagnosis, (2) were continuously enrolled in Medicare Parts A and B in the year of, before, and after they were diagnosed,[9] and (3) received a prostate biopsy on the same day as or within 1 year prior to their diagnosis.[10] We then analyzed prostate cancer–related claims from the Medicare Part B Carrier and hospital outpatient files to determine what types of treatments these beneficiaries received from their diagnosis date through 1 year after that date.[11] We used the provider who performed a beneficiary's prostate biopsy that was nearest to his date of diagnosis as a proxy for the provider who referred the beneficiary for treatment. We classified referring providers as self-referring if they were the performing provider on a claim that was paid to a self-referring provider group in the year of, before, or after a beneficiary's prostate cancer diagnosis. All other providers were considered non-self-referring. Similarly, we classified providers as belonging to a limited-specialty group if they were the performing provider on a claim that was paid to a limited-specialty provider group in the year of, before, or after a beneficiary's prostate cancer diagnosis. If a provider did not belong to a limited-specialty group, we considered the provider to belong to a multispecialty group.

To assess the possibility that beneficiary characteristics affected the types of treatments for which self-referring and non-self-referring providers referred their prostate cancer patients, we examined beneficiaries' (1) age at the time they were diagnosed with prostate cancer, (2) geographic location (i.e., urban or rural), and (3) health, including clinical characteristics of prostate cancers for a subset of beneficiaries who lived in New York. We determined a beneficiary's age at diagnosis using a beneficiary's date of birth and the date on which he was diagnosed with prostate cancer. We defined urban settings as metropolitan statistical areas, a geographic entity defined by the Office of Management and Budget as a core urban area of 50,000 or more population. We used rural-urban commuting area codes—a Census tract– based classification scheme that utilizes the standard Bureau of Census Urbanized Area and Urban Cluster definitions in combination with work-commuting information to characterize all of the nation's Census tracts regarding their rural and urban status—to identify beneficiaries as living in metropolitan statistical areas.[12] We considered all other settings to be rural. We used CMS's risk score file to identify average risk score, which serves as a proxy for beneficiary health status. For a subset of beneficiaries who lived in New York, we obtained clinical information on the beneficiaries' prostate cancer—including information used to determine whether the localized cancer was low, intermediate, or high risk—from the New York State Cancer Registry.[13] To establish whether a prostate cancer was low, intermediate, or high risk, we used a beneficiary's Gleason score, prostate-specific antigen (PSA), and tumor stage from the New York State Cancer Registry.[14] The results of the New York analysis are not generalizable to the entire Medicare population.

We also determined whether the percentage of a provider's prostate cancer patients referred for IMRT changed after providers began to self-refer. Specifically, we identified a group of providers, which we called "switchers," that did not self-refer in 2006 or 2007 but began to self-refer in either 2008 or 2009. We then calculated the change in the percentage of switchers' patients referred for IMRT and other treatments among those diagnosed with prostate cancer in 2007 and 2009. We then compared the change among switchers to the change experienced by providers that did not change whether or not they self-referred IMRT services from 2007 to 2009. Specifically, we compared the change in the percentage of switchers' prostate cancer patients they referred for IMRT to the percentage of patients referred for IMRT by (1) self-referring providers—providers that self-referred in 2007, 2008, and 2009 and either self-referred or did not bill Medicare in 2006 and 2010 and (2) non-self-referring providers—providers that did not self-refer in 2007, 2008, and 2009 and either did not self-refer or did not bill Medicare in 2006 and 2010.15

We took several steps to ensure that the data used to produce this report were sufficiently reliable. Specifically, we assessed the reliability of the CMS data we used by interviewing officials responsible for overseeing these data sources, including CMS and Medicare contractor officials. We also reviewed relevant documentation and examined the data for obvious errors, such as missing values and values outside of expected ranges. We determined that the data were sufficiently reliable for the purposes of our study.

We conducted this performance audit from May 2010 through July 2013 in accordance with generally accepted government auditing standards. Those standards require that we plan and perform the audit to obtain sufficient, appropriate evidence to provide a reasonable basis for our findings and conclusions based on our audit objectives. We believe that the evidence obtained provides a reasonable basis for our findings and conclusions based on our audit objectives.

APPENDIX II: CHANGE IN PROSTATE CANCER–RELATED IMRT SERVICES AND EXPENDITURES BY SETTING

Medicare prostate cancer–related intensity-modulated radiation therapy (IMRT) utilization varied substantially between settings (see figure 4). From 2006 through 2010, utilization grew at an annual rate of 10 percent in physician offices, whereas there was almost no growth in the hospital outpatient department. Moreover, while the utilization of prostate cancer– related IMRT services in the hospital outpatient department was nearly the same in 2006 as it was in 2010, utilization in this setting actually peaked in 2007 and declined thereafter.

Total prostate cancer–related IMRT expenditures grew from $589 million to $698 million over our study period, but growth rates varied by setting (see figure 5). In contrast to the growth in utilization, expenditures increased faster for services performed in hospital outpatient departments than those performed in physician offices—7 percent and 3 percent annual growth rates, respectively. This is due to the fact that reimbursement rates for IMRT services have been increasing for services performed in hospital outpatient departments and declining for those performed in physician offices.

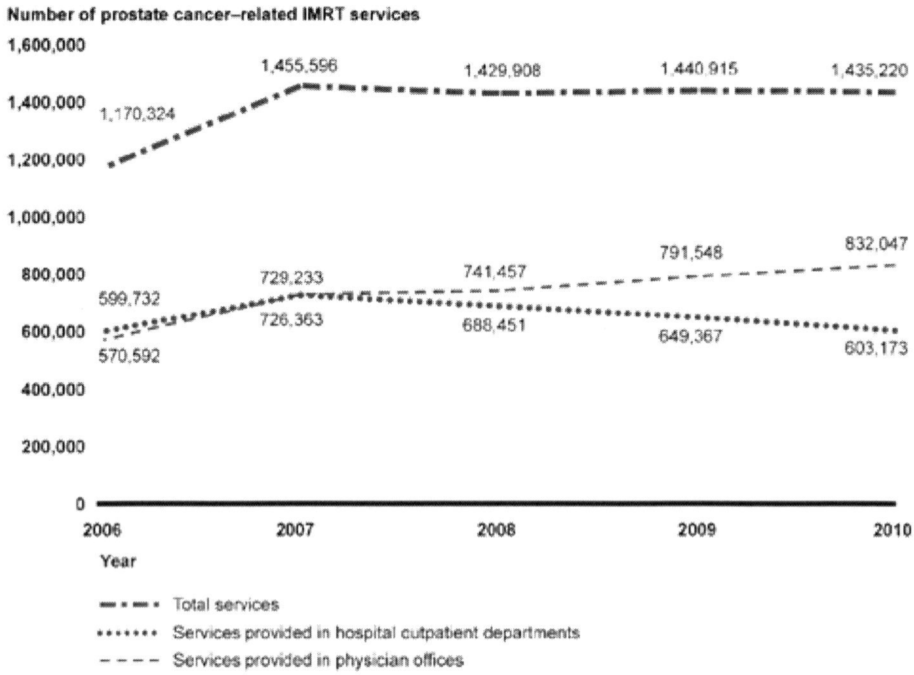

Source: GAO analysis of CMS data.

Figure 4. Number of Medicare Prostate Cancer–Related IMRT Services by Setting, 2006-2010.

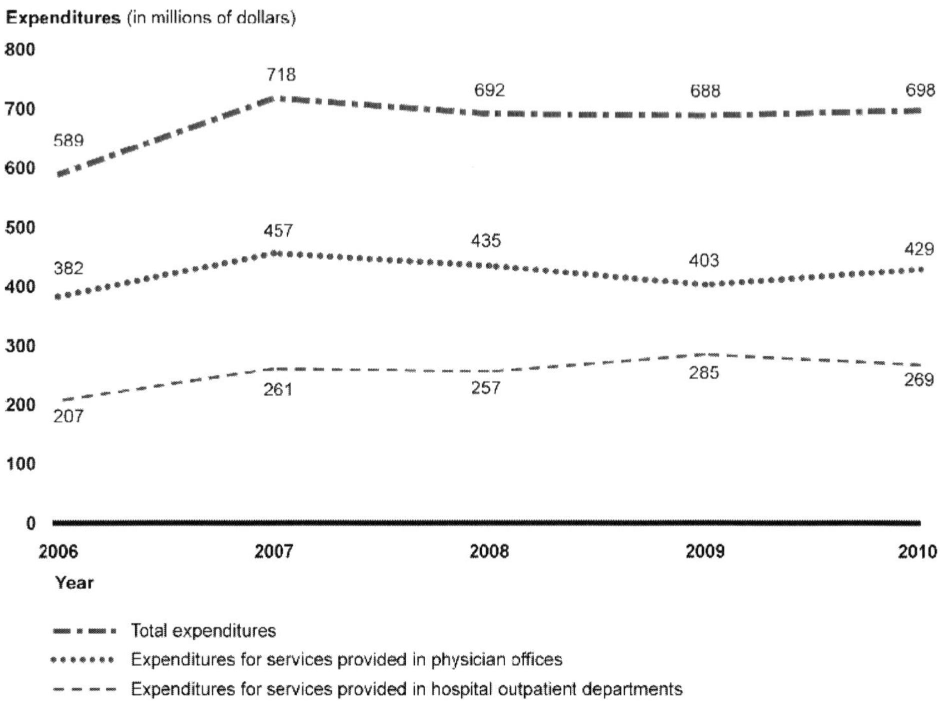

Source: GAO analysis of CMS data.

Figure 5. Expenditures for Medicare Prostate Cancer–Related IMRT Services by Setting, 2006-2010.

APPENDIX III: DISCRETE PROSTATE CANCER TREATMENT CATEGORIES

The higher percentage of patients that self-referring Medicare providers referred for intensity-modulated radiation therapy (IMRT) compared to non-self-referring providers was due to self-referring providers referring their patients for IMRT only and IMRT in conjunction with hormone therapy more often (see table 4). Including all combinations, self-referring and non-self-referring providers referred nearly equal percentages of their patients for a combination of treatments—27 percent and 26 percent, respectively.

Table 4. Percentage of Self-Referring and Non-Self-Referring Providers' Medicare Patients Referred for a Given Treatment or Combination of Treatments after Diagnosis of Prostate Cancer in 2009

Prostate cancer treatment	Percentage of non-self-referring providers' patients referred for a given treatment (N=48,298)	Percentage of self-referring providers' patients referred for a given treatment (N=9,991)	Percentage point difference
IMRT only	12.8%	27.0%	14.2
IMRT and radical prostatectomy	1.2	0.9	-0.3
IMRT and brachytherapy	4.7	2.6	-2.0
IMRT and hormone therapy	13.2	20.1	6.9
Active surveillance	22.9	21.0	-1.9
Radical prostatectomy only	15.5	11.5	-4.0
Radical prostatectomy and hormone therapy	1.1	0.6	-0.5
Hormone therapy only	11.4	7.7	-3.8
Brachytherapy only	6.5	3.5	-3.0
Brachytherapy and hormone therapy	2.2	0.7	-1.5
Other treatments only[a]	4.4	2.5	-2.0
Other treatments and hormone therapy	1.3	0.6	-0.7
Three-dimensional conformal radiation therapy(3D-CRT) / other external beam radiation therapy (EBRT) only	0.2	0.0	-0.1
3D-CRT / other EBRT and hormone therapy	0.3	0.1	-0.2
Other combinations[b]	2.2	1.1	-1.1

Source: GAO analysis of CMS data.

Notes: Percentages do not sum to 100 percent due to rounding. Beneficiaries were sorted into "IMRT and brachytherapy" and "IMRT and radical prostatectomy" if they received IMRT plus the treatment or IMRT plus the treatment and hormone therapy. Beneficiaries sorted into "IMRT and hormone therapy" did not receive any other treatments. Men were considered to have received a combination of therapies if they received at least one service from two or more different types of treatments. We did not differentiate on the basis of the order of different treatment combinations or the duration of treatments.

[a]"Other treatments" consists of cryoablation, stereotactic body radiotherapy / stereotactic radiosurgery, and proton therapy.

[b]"Other combinations" includes any combination of treatments that does not have a separate category, such as 3D-CRT / other EBRT and brachytherapy.

APPENDIX IV: DISTRIBUTION OF PROSTATE CANCER TREATMENTS BY AGE

While self-referring Medicare providers were more likely to refer their prostate cancer patients for intensity-modulated radiation therapy (IMRT) regardless of age, the type of treatment they were less likely to refer their patients for varied based on the age of the beneficiary (see table 5). For instance, among beneficiaries 80 years of age or older at the time they were diagnosed with prostate cancer, self-referring providers were less likely to refer their prostate cancer patients for hormone therapy only, active surveillance, and brachytherapy compared to non-self-referring providers. In contrast, among beneficiaries 66 to 69 years old, nearly the entire difference between self-referring and non-self-referring providers was due to self-referring providers referring a smaller percentage of their prostate cancer patients for a radical prostatectomy or brachytherapy.

Table 5. Percentage of Self-Referring and Non-Self-Referring Providers' Medicare Patients Referred for a Given Treatment after a Diagnosis of Prostate Cancer in 2009 by Age of Beneficiary

	Age category (in years)							
	Percentage of non-self-referring providers' patients referred for a given treatment by age category (years)				Percentage of self-referring providers' patients referred for a given treatment by age category (years)			
Prostate cancer treatment	66-69 (N=12,988)	70-74 (N=16,710)	75-79 (N=11,025)	≥80 (N=7,575)	66-69 (N=2,636)	70-74 (N=3,434)	75-79 (N=2,340)	≥80 (N=1,581)
IMRT	29.1%	36.3%	40.7%	25.7%	46.6%	54.5%	60.1%	41.8%
Active surveillance	18.1	20.7	25.9	31.4	16.1	20.1	22.4	29.0
Radical prostatectomy	35.8	20.5	5.1	0.6	28.3	14.1	3.2	0.4
Hormone therapy only	4.1	6.2	11.8	35.0	2.7	3.9	7.1	25.1
Brachytherapy	15.5	16.6	14.4	5.2	8.9	8.4	6.2	2.0
Other treatments[a]	5.2	6.7	7.4	3.9	3.2	3.3	3.6	2.7
Three-dimensional conformal radiation therapy / other external beam radiation therapy	2.2	2.7	2.9	1.8	1.0	1.1	1.3	1.0

Source: GAO analysis of CMS data.

Notes: Treatment categories do not sum to 100 percent because, with the exception of active surveillance and hormone therapy only, the categories are not mutually exclusive.

[a]"Other treatments" consists of cryoablation, stereotactic body radiotherapy/ stereotactic radiosurgery, and proton therapy.

APPENDIX V: CHANGE IN PROSTATE CANCER TREATMENT PATTERNS OVER TIME FOR DIFFERENT TYPES OF PROVIDERS

The increased percentage of Medicare patients referred by switchers for intensity-modulated radiation therapy (IMRT) was accompanied by a decrease in the percentage of patients referred for several other treatments, especially brachytherapy (see table 6). Some of the changes in the percentage of patients referred by switchers for a given treatment were consistent with the patterns for other types of providers—such as in the case of three-dimensional conformal radiation therapy (3D-CRT) / other external beam radiation therapy (EBRT)—while some of the other changes were not.

Table 6. Change in the Percentage of Medicare Prostate Cancer Patients Providers Referred for a Given Treatment after a Diagnosis of Prostate Cancer in 2007 or 2009

Prostate cancer treatment	Type of provider	Percentage of providers' patients referred for a given treatment among beneficiaries diagnosed in 2007	Percentage of providers' patients referred for a given treatment among beneficiaries diagnosed in 2009	Percentage point change from 2007 to 2009	Percentage more orless likely providerswere to refer patientsfor a given treatment in2009 compared to 2007
IMRT	Non-self-referring	31.4%	33.1%	1.7	5.5%
	Self-referring	55.7	52.9	-2.8	-5.1
	Switcher	37.0	54.2	17.2	46.6
Active surveillance	Non-self-referring	19.3	22.6	3.3	17.3
	Self-referring	17.3	20.7	3.4	19.6
	Switcher	18.1	20.1	2.0	11.2
Brachytherapy	Non-self-referring	17.6	14.4	-3.2	-18.2
	Self-referring	4.7	2.3	-2.5	-52.4
	Switcher	20.7	9.9	-10.8	-52.2
Radical prostatectomy	Non-self-referring	16.6	18.0	1.4	8.5
	Self-referring	13.1	15.1	2.0	15.7
	Switcher	13.0	11.1	-1.9	-14.5
Hormone therapy only	Non-self-referring	14.3	11.6	-2.7	-18.6
	Self-referring	8.6	7.9	-0.7	-8.6
	Switcher	13.1	8.0	-5.1	-39.1
3D-CRT / other EBRT	Non-self-referring	5.0	2.5	-2.5	-50.4
	Self-referring	0.8	0.7	-0.1	-14.3
	Switcher	4.0	1.3	-2.7	-68.7
Other treatments[a]	Non-self-referring	5.7	6.3	0.6	10.8
	Self-referring	1.8	2.5	0.7	38.3
	Switcher	4.8	1.9	-2.8	-59.7

Source: GAO analysis of CMS data.

Notes: Treatment categories for each type of provider do not sum to 100 percent because, with the exception of active surveillance and hormone therapy only, the categories are not mutually exclusive. In 2007, switchers, self-referring providers, and non-self-referring providers referred 4,903, 1,776, and 42,471 prostate cancer patients for treatment, respectively. In 2009, switchers, self-referring providers, and non-self-referring providers referred 4,156, 1,244, and 34,107 prostate cancer patients for treatment, respectively. Because some treatments were relatively rare, some provider type, treatment group, and year categories, such as patients referred for 3D-CRT / other EBRT by self-referring providers in 2009, have relatively few beneficiaries. However, the results of this analysis are consistent with the trends observed when referral patterns for self-referring and non-self-referring providers were studied for all beneficiaries diagnosed in 2007 and 2009.

[a]"Other treatments" consists of cryoablation, stereotactic body radiotherapy / stereotactic radiosurgery, and proton therapy.

End Notes

[1] Providers in our analysis that could self-refer could include physicians and other providers, such as nurse practitioners and physician assistants.

[2] Compliance with the physician self-referral law, commonly known as the Stark law, is outside the scope of this report. The Stark law prohibits physicians from making referrals for certain designated health services paid for by Medicare, to entities with which the physicians or immediate family members have a financial relationship, unless the arrangement complies with a specified exception, such as in-office ancillary services. 42 U.S.C. § 1395nn(b)(2). The requirements of the in-office ancillary services exception are found at 42 C.F.R. § 411.355(b) (2012).

[3] For example, see Benjamin P. Falit, Cary P. Gross, and Kenneth B. Roberts, "Integrated Prostate Cancer Centers and Over-Utilization of IMRT: A Close Look at Fee-For-Service Medicine in Radiation Oncology," *International Journal of Radiation Oncology • Biology • Physics* 76, no. 5 (April 2010): 1285-88.

[4] For instance, for a subset of localized prostate cancers that are low risk, IMRT, brachytherapy, and a radical prostatectomy are all among the treatments considered appropriate. According to the National Cancer Institute, 81 percent of men who were diagnosed with prostate cancer from 2002 through 2008 in 18 geographic areas that provided cancer data to the National Cancer Institute were diagnosed with localized prostate cancer, while the rest were diagnosed at an unknown stage (3 percent) or after the cancer had spread regionally (12 percent) or distantly (4 percent). See http://seer.cancer.gov/statfacts/html/prost.html, accessed December 18, 2012.

[5] IMRT delivery codes represent individual treatment sessions during which patients receive radiation. In addition to receiving radiation, patients receive several different types of services during a course of IMRT. Our analysis of self-referred prostate cancer–related IMRT services is limited to those services performed in physician offices. We focused on this setting because our work showed rapid growth in this setting compared to hospital outpatient departments and because the financial incentive for providers to self-refer is most direct when the service is performed in a physician office. Services performed by non-self-referring groups in the physician office setting could include services provided in places such as freestanding cancer centers. Throughout this report, we refer to services billed through the Carrier file as services performed in physician offices.

[6] An indicator or "flag" could be, for example, a modifier that a provider lists on a claim to indicate that a service is self-referred. Providers currently use modifiers to provide additional information about a service to CMS.

[7] Providers could have a financial relationship with the same entity if, for example, they are part of the same group practice.

[8] We defined urban areas as metropolitan statistical areas, a geographic entity defined by the Office of Management and Budget as a core urban area of 50,000 or more population; all other settings were considered rural.

[9] National Cancer Institute. See http://seer.cancer accessed December 18, 2012. Skin cancer is the most common form of cancer.

[10] Men can also receive a combination of therapies, such as brachytherapy combined with EBRT.

[11] National Comprehensive Cancer Network, *NCCN Clinical Practice Guidelines in Oncology (NCCN GuidelinesTM): Prostate Cancer* (June 2011).

[12] Institute for Clinical and Economic Review, "Management Options for Low-Risk Prostate Cancer: A Report on Comparative Effectiveness and Value" (Sept. 16, 2009).

[13] Steven B. Zelladt et al., "Why Do Men Choose One Treatment over Another? A Review of Patient Decision Making for Localized Prostate Cancer," *Cancer* 106, no. 9 (May 1, 2006): 1865-74.

[14] Vahakn B. Shahinian, Yong-Fang Kuo, and Scott M. Gilbert, "Reimbursement Policy and Androgen-Deprivation Therapy for Prostate Cancer," *The New England Journal of Medicine* 363, no. 19 (Nov. 4, 2010): 1822-32.

[15] A physician with an ownership or investment interest in a hospital and who is a member of that hospital's medical staff is required to disclose this financial interest when referring patients to that hospital under an exception to the general prohibition on Medicare self-referral (Stark law). According to Physician Hospitals of America, an advocacy group for physician-owned hospitals, approximately 265 hospitals—or less than 5 percent of all hospitals—were physician-owned as of July 2012. See 42 C.F.R. § 411.362 (2012) for more information on additional requirements concerning physician ownership and investment in hospitals under the Stark law. The Patient Protection and Affordable Care Act (PPACA) created a new disclosure requirement for physicians who self-refer certain other in-office ancillary services under the Stark Law. Pub. L. No. 111-148, § 6003, 124 Stat. 119, 697(2010). Specifically, referring physicians for certain advanced imaging services are required to inform their patients in writing at the time of the referral that the patient may obtain the service from another entity and provide the patients with a list of providers who furnish the service in the area in which the patient resides. 42 U.S.C. § 13955nn(b)(2). No such requirement exists for physicians who self-refer IMRT services. CMS noted in the preamble to the final rule detailing this disclosure requirement that the agency does not have the authority to expand the disclosure requirements to services other than the radiology services referenced in PPACA. Medicare Program; Payment Policies Under the Physician Fee Schedule and Other Revisions to Part B for CY 2011, 75 Fed. Reg. 73,170, 73,444 (Nov. 29, 2010).

[16] These payment rates are those hospitals receive under the Hospital Outpatient Prospective Payment System. Not all hospitals are paid under this system.

[17] These expenditures do not include the payment reductions that may result from implementation of the Budget Control Act of 2011. Pub. L. No. 112-25, 125 Stat. 240.

[18] The technical component is intended to cover the cost of performing a test, including the costs for equipment, supplies, and nonphysician staff.

[19] Episodes of IMRT for prostate cancer include other services such as a radiotherapy dose plan, weekly management services, and weekly radiation physics consultations.

[20] For instance, see: Matthew R. Cooperberg et al., "Primary treatments for clinically localised prostate cancer: a comprehensive lifetime cost utility analysis," *BJU International* 111, no. 3 (March 2013): 437-50; or Chirag Shah et al., "Brachytherapy provides comparable outcomes and improved cost-effectiveness in the treatment of low/intermediate prostate cancer," *Brachytherapy* 11 (2012): 441-45.

[21] P. L. Nguyen et al., "Cost implications of the rapid adoption of newer technologies for treating prostate cancer," *Journal of Clinical Oncology*, 29, no. 12 (2011): 1517-24. Because Medicare beneficiaries often face cost-sharing requirements, more expensive treatments likely lead to higher beneficiary costs.

[22] To determine the effect of the payment reduction, we calculated the cost of a course of IMRT to treat prostate cancer using 2013 Medicare reimbursement rates and previously published methodologies. For an example of a methodology used, see Andre Konski et al., "Using Decision Analysis to Determine the Cost-Effectiveness of Intensity-Modulated Radiation Therapy in the Treatment of Intermediate Risk Prostate Cancer," *International Journal of Radiation Oncology • Biology • Physics* 66, no. 2 (2006): 408-15.

[23] Specifically, our analysis of the distribution of treatments among men newly diagnosed with prostate cancer indicates that 33.7 percent and 36.8 percent of men diagnosed with prostate cancer in 2007 and 2009, respectively, were referred for IMRT.

[24] As a result of increased enrollment in Medicare Advantage, the number of Medicare FFS beneficiaries aged 65 and older decreased from 2006 to 2010, going from approximately 27.6 million to 26.4 million.

[25] In our analysis of the distribution of treatments among men newly diagnosed with prostate cancer, we found a 19 percent decrease in the number of Medicare FFS beneficiaries who were diagnosed with prostate cancer and met our other inclusion criteria in 2009 compared to 2007—58,289 and 71,834, respectively. In accordance with that, the number of prostate biopsies provided to Medicare FFS beneficiaries, which some researchers have used as a proxy for prostate cancer diagnoses, stayed relatively flat from 2006 to 2007 but then decreased by approximately 20 percent from 2007 through 2010. Others have also noted a decline in reported prostate cancer incidence over a similar period. For instance, see: David H. Howard, "Declines in Prostate Cancer Incidence After Changes in Screening Recommendations," *Archives of Internal Medicine* 172, no. 16 (Sept. 10, 2012): 1267-68.

[26] Bruce L. Jacobs et al., "Growth of High-Cost Intensity-Modulated Radiotherapy for Prostate Cancer Raises Concerns About Overuse," *Health Affairs* 31, no. 4 (April 2012): 750-59.

[27] In 2010, urologists performed approximately 89.1 percent of office visits billed under limited-specialty groups, compared to 5.7 percent for multispecialty groups. Additionally, the average number of specialties that billed office visits under limited-specialty groups in 2010 was 3.3, compared to 36.2 for multispecialty groups.

[28] Other than IMRT, the only type of treatment for which self-referring providers did not refer a lower percentage of their prostate cancer patients compared to non-self-referring providers was proton therapy.

[29] Because only a small percentage of beneficiaries were referred by providers who belonged to a multispecialty group, we combined beneficiaries diagnosed with prostate cancer in 2007 or 2009. Of that population, approximately 92 percent were referred by a provider who belonged to a limited-specialty group, compared to 8 percent who were referred by a provider who belonged to a multispecialty group.

[30] Approximately 84 percent of self-referring providers' prostate cancer patients lived in urban areas compared to approximately 68 percent of non-self-referring providers' patients.

[31] A beneficiary's risk score is a proxy for health status and is equivalent to the ratio of expected health care expenditures for the beneficiary under Medicare FFS relative to the average health care expenditures for all Medicare FFS beneficiaries. For example, a beneficiary with a risk score of 1.05 would have expected expenditures that were 5 percent higher than an average Medicare FFS beneficiary.

[32] Self-referring providers were also 43 percent more likely to refer their patients for IMRT compared to non-self-referring providers for patients who could not be assigned a risk category. Because the New York State Cancer Registry contains some cancer characteristics obtained after patients received treatment, we also reran this analysis twice after restricting the population to patients (1) for whom the extent of the cancer was determined before treatment and (2) who did not receive a radical prostatectomy. For both of these analyses, the results were similar to the original analysis—self-referring providers were between 25 percent and 87 percent more likely to refer their patients for IMRT compared to non-self-referring providers, depending on whether the cancer was low, intermediate, or high risk.

[33] While the difference between self-referring and non-self-referring providers narrowed, non-self-referring providers were still more likely to refer their patients with intermediate- and high-risk prostate cancer for brachytherapy compared to self-referring providers. This includes brachytherapy as a sole treatment or brachytherapy received in combination with another treatment, such as a form of EBRT.

[34] We used clinical information from the New York State Cancer Registry because such information is not available on Medicare claims, and we determined that the geographic areas included in another common source of such information—Surveillance Epidemiology and End Results (SEER) data—did not sufficiently overlap with areas in which IMRT self-referral was prevalent during our study period.

[35] Thomas L. Jang et al., "Physician Visits Prior to Treatment for Clinically Localized Prostate Cancer," *Archives of Internal Medicine* 172, no.5 (March 8, 2010): 440-450.

End Notes for Appendix I

[1] We also used the Part B National Summary Data Files to track the total number of prostate biopsies from 2006 through 2010. The Medicare Part B Carrier File contains final action Medicare Part B claims for noninstitutional providers, such as physicians. The Medicare hospital outpatient file contains final action, fee-for-service claims data submitted by institutional outpatient providers, such as hospital outpatient departments.

[2] Medicare expenditure amounts for these codes include beneficiary cost sharing throughout this report. IMRT delivery codes represent individual treatment sessions during which patients receive radiation. In addition to receiving radiation, patients receive several different types of services during a course of IMRT.

[3] Our analysis of self-referred prostate cancer–related IMRT services is limited to those services performed in physician offices. We focused on this setting because our work showed rapid growth in this setting compared to hospital outpatient departments and because the financial incentive for providers to self-refer is most direct when the service is performed in a physician office. We refer to services billed through the Carrier file as services performed in physician offices.

[4] An indicator or "flag" could be, for example, a modifier that a provider lists on a claim to indicate that a service is self-referred. Providers currently use modifiers to provide additional information about a service to CMS.

[5] From 2006 through 2010, beneficiaries could receive multiple episodes of prostate cancer–related IMRT. We defined an episode of IMRT as a contiguous group of IMRT services not separated by more than 7 days. If a beneficiary had more than one prostate-cancer related IMRT episode over the course of our study, we classified each episode as self-referred or non-self-referred separately.

[6] Respectively, these restrictions were made to ensure that we (1) did not classify groups as self-referring on the basis of a small percentage of the IMRT episodes they provided, (2) classified groups on the basis of the predominant way in which the group practiced, and (3) had an adequate number of IMRT episodes to accurately categorize groups.

[7] Services performed by non-self-referring groups in the physician office setting could include services provided in places such as freestanding cancer centers.

[8] Self-referral occurs when providers refer their patients to entities—such as themselves or a group practice—in which they or a member of their families has a financial relationship. We used TINs to identify financial relationships between the provider who performed the prostate biopsy and the provider(s) who administered IMRT.

[9] This requirement includes not being enrolled in Medicare Advantage in the year of, before, or after a beneficiary's prostate cancer diagnosis.

[10] These restrictions removed beneficiaries for whom the diagnosis date could have been unrelated to when they were actually diagnosed with prostate cancer. For instance, a 65-year-old beneficiary could have been diagnosed with prostate cancer before aging onto Medicare, and, therefore, the claims-based diagnosis date could have represented when the beneficiary became eligible for Medicare rather than when he was first diagnosed.

[11] We did not determine whether treatments were curative or palliative. We also did not differentiate on the basis of the order of different treatment combinations or the duration of treatments. A prostate cancer patient was considered to have undergone active surveillance if he—in addition to meeting the general inclusion criteria—did not receive a service indicating that he received any other prostate cancer treatment within one year of diagnosis.

[12] We considered a location with a rural-urban commuting area code of 1.0, 1.1, 2.0, 2.1, or 3.0 to be a metropolitan statistical area.

[13] This analysis includes beneficiaries who were diagnosed with prostate cancer in either 2007 or 2009.

[14] Such information is not available on Medicare claims. Researchers commonly use the National Cancer Institute's Surveillance Epidemiology and End Results (SEER) data to obtain clinical information about Medicare patients who were diagnosed with cancer. We did not use SEER data because we examined treatments received by men diagnosed with prostate cancer in 2007 and 2009, and, in 2007, IMRT self-referral was concentrated in states not included in SEER data. Respectively, low , intermediate , and high risk prostate cancers were defined as follows: T1-T2a, Gleason score 2-6, and PSA < 10 ng/ml; T2bT2c, Gleason score 7, or PSA 10-20 ng/ml; and T3a, Gleason score 8-10, or PSA > 20 ng/ml.

[15] For this analysis and our analysis of all providers who referred a Medicare beneficiary in our study who was diagnosed with prostate cancer in 2007 or 2009, we counted IMRT and other treatments regardless of the setting in which they were performed.

In: Physician Self-Referrals
Editor: Louise Hamilton
ISBN: 978-1-63463-444-1

Chapter 3

MEDICARE: ACTION NEEDED TO ADDRESS HIGHER USE OF ANATOMIC PATHOLOGY SERVICES BY PROVIDERS WHO SELF-REFER*

United States Government Accountability Office

WHY GAO DID THIS STUDY

Questions have been raised about selfreferral's role in Medicare Part B expenditures' rapid growth. Self-referral occurs when providers refer patients to entities in which they or their family members have a financial interest. Services that can be self-referred under certain circumstances include anatomic pathology—the preparation and examination of tissue samples to diagnose disease. GAO was asked to examine the prevalence of anatomic pathology self-referral and its effect on Medicare spending. This report examines (1) trends in the number of and expenditures for self-referred and non-self-referred anatomic pathology services, (2) how provision of these services may differ on the basis of whether providers self-refer, and (3) implications of self-referral for Medicare spending. GAO analyzed Medicare Part B claims data from 2004 through 2010 and interviewed officials from the Centers for Medicare & Medicaid Services (CMS) and other stakeholders. GAO developed a claims-based approach to identify self-referred services because Medicare claims lack such an indicator.

WHAT GAO RECOMMENDS

CMS should identify self-referred anatomic pathology services and address their higher use. The Department of Health and Human Services, which oversees CMS, agreed with GAO's recommendation that CMS address higher use of self-referral through a payment approach, but disagreed with GAO's other two recommendations to identify self-referred

* This is an edited, reformatted and augmented version of a United States Government Accountability Office publication, No. GAO-13-445, dated June 2013.

services and address their higher use. GAO believes the recommended actions could result in Medicare savings.

WHAT GAO FOUND

Self-referred anatomic pathology services increased at a faster rate than nonself-referred services from 2004 to 2010. During this period, the number of self-referred anatomic pathology services more than doubled, growing from 1.06 million services to about 2.26 million services, while non-self-referred services grew about 38 percent, from about 5.64 million services to about 7.77 million services. Similarly, the growth rate of expenditures for self-referred anatomic pathology services was higher than for non-self-referred services. Three provider specialties—dermatology, gastroenterology, and urology—accounted for 90 percent of referrals for self-referred anatomic pathology services in 2010.

Referrals for anatomic pathology services by dermatologists, gastroenterologists, and urologists substantially increased the year after they began to self-refer. Providers that began self-referring in 2009—referred to as switchers—had increases in anatomic pathology services that ranged on average from 14.0 percent to 58.5 percent in 2010 compared to 2008, the year before they began self-referring, across these provider specialties. In comparison, increases in anatomic pathology referrals for providers who continued to self-refer or never self-referred services during this period were much lower. Thus, the increase in anatomic pathology referrals for switchers was not due to a general increase in use of these services among all providers. GAO's examination of all providers that referred an anatomic pathology service in 2010 showed that self-referring providers of the specialties we examined referred more services on average than non-self referring providers. Differences in referral for these services generally persisted after accounting for geography and patient characteristics such as health status and diagnosis. These analyses suggest that financial incentives for self-referring providers were likely a major factor driving the increase in referrals.

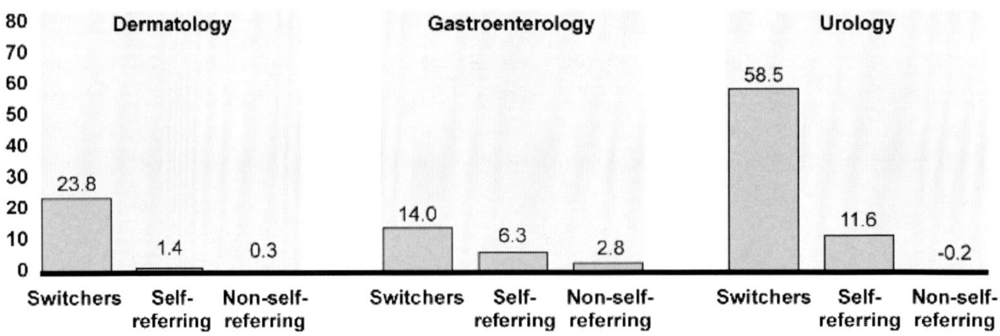

Source: GAO analysis of CMS data.

Note: Switchers are providers that did not self-refer in 2007 or 2008, but did self-refer in 2009 and 2010.

Percentage Change in Medicare Anatomic Pathology Services by Provider Specialty, 2008 to 2010.

GAO estimates that in 2010, self-referring providers likely referred over 918,000 more anatomic pathology services than if they had performed biopsy procedures at the same rate as and referred the same number of services per biopsy procedure as non-self-referring providers. These additional referrals for anatomic pathology services cost Medicare about $69 million. To the extent that these additional referrals were unnecessary, avoiding them could result in savings to Medicare and beneficiaries, as they share in the cost of services.

ABBREVIATIONS

AADA	American Academy of Dermatology Association
AGA	American Gastroenterological Association
AUA	American Urological Association
CAP	College of American Pathologists
CMS	Centers for Medicare & Medicaid Services
HHS	Department of Health and Human Services
FFS	fee-for-service
HCPCS	Healthcare Common Procedure Coding System
ICD-9-CM	International Classification of Diseases, Ninth Revision, Clinical Modification
NPI	national provider identifier
OIG	Office of Inspector General
PC	professional component
TC	technical component
TIN	taxpayer identification number

* * *

June 24, 2013

Congressional Requesters:

Expenditures for Medicare Part B services—which include physician and other outpatient services—have grown rapidly, increasing annually at 5.9 percent, on average, from 2007 through 2011. In comparison, the national economy grew by less than half that rate during the same time period. Some policymakers have raised questions about the growth in Part B spending, including the extent to which this growth may be attributable to financial incentives that exist for physicians to self-refer certain services. Self-referral occurs when providers refer their patients for services delivered by entities—such as themselves or a group practice—with which the providers or an immediate family member has a financial relationship. While federal law generally prohibits self-referral under Medicare, there are exceptions for certain services and arrangements.[1]

Among the Medicare diagnostic and therapeutic services that may be self-referred under one of these exceptions are anatomic pathology services, in which physicians trained as pathologists prepare and examine tissue samples and other specimens to diagnose disease and guide patient care.[2] Providers from an array of physician specialties, including dermatology, urology, and gastroenterology, may self-refer the preparation of a patient's tissue for examination, the examination of this tissue to make a diagnosis, or both. Proponents of self-referral contend that arrangements in which physicians have laboratories in their offices allow providers to make rapid diagnoses and improve coordination of care. In 2010, expenditures for anatomic pathology services under the Medicare physician fee schedule—the payment system used to determine fees for physician-billed services in Medicare fee-for-service (FFS)—totaled $1.94 billon.

While we and other federal agencies have reported on physician self-referral, only a series of studies by the Department of Health and Human Services (HHS) Office of the Inspector General (OIG) has focused explicitly on how self-referral may affect the provision of anatomic pathology services.[3] Specifically, in 2007, HHS OIG issued three studies that examined self-referral of anatomic pathology services among three urology practices. The HHS OIG found that, for all three practices, utilization of anatomic pathology services increased after the practice began to self-refer.

You asked us to examine the prevalence of self-referral of anatomic pathology services and Medicare spending for these services.[4] In this report, we examine (1) trends in the number of and expenditures for self-referred and non-self-referred anatomic pathology services from 2004 through 2010, (2) how the provision of anatomic pathology services may differ for providers who self-refer when compared with other providers, and (3) the implications of self-referral for Medicare spending on anatomic pathology services.

To identify trends in the number of and expenditures for self-referred and non-self-referred anatomic pathology services, we analyzed claims from the Medicare Part B Carrier File for 2004 through 2010. Because there is no indicator or "flag" on Medicare claims that identifies whether or not services were self-referred, we developed a claims-based methodology to identify services as either self-referred or non-self-referred.[5] Specifically, we classified services as self-referred if the provider that referred the beneficiary for an anatomic pathology service and the provider that performed the anatomic pathology service were identical or had a financial relationship with the same entity.[6] We focused our review of anatomic pathology services and service components to services with a Healthcare Common Procedure Coding System (HCPCS) code 88305, which is the code for anatomic pathology services related to the examination of tissue samples taken through biopsy procedures.[7] About 66 percent of the $1.94 billion in expenditures for anatomic pathology services in 2010 were associated with HCPCS code 88305. (We also reviewed services with HCPCS codes 88312, 88313, and 88342—special stains—which are used in conjunction with anatomic pathology services to assist providers in making a diagnosis. See app. I for our analysis related to special stains.) We limited the universe for this portion of our analysis to those anatomic pathology services performed in a provider's office or in an independent clinical laboratory.[8] We focused on these settings because the financial incentive for providers to self-refer is most direct when the service is performed in a physician office. Further, we limited our analysis to self-referral of the preparation of these services, because we could determine that the services were performed in a physician's office or independent laboratory.[9] We used the claims to identify trends in the number and proportion of self-referred and non-selfreferred anatomic pathology services performed from 2004 through 2010, the expenditures for these services from 2004 through 2010, and the proportion of self-referred and non-self-referred anatomic pathology services by provider specialty for 2004 and 2010. To determine expenditures, we used the allowed charges variable from the Medicare Part B Carrier File, which includes the amounts paid by Medicare and the beneficiary.

To determine how the provision of anatomic pathology services may differ for providers who self-refer when compared with other providers, we performed two separate analyses. First, we compared the provision—that is, the number of referrals made—of anatomic pathology services by self-referring providers and non-self-referring providers in 2010, disaggregated by provider size (i.e., the number of Medicare beneficiaries seen by the provider), provider specialty, geography (i.e., urban or rural) and patient characteristics. [10] Second, we determined the extent to which the number of anatomic pathology referrals made by providers changed after the providers began to self-refer. Specifically, we identified a group of providers who began to self-refer anatomic pathology services in 2009 and calculated the change in the number of anatomic pathology referrals the providers made from 2008 (i.e., the year before they began self-referring) through 2010 (i.e., the year after they began self-referring).[11] We then compared this change to the change made by (1) providers who self-referred anatomic pathology services over this time period and (2) providers who did not self-refer services over the time period.

To determine the implications of self-referral for Medicare spending on anatomic pathology services, we summed the number of and expenditures for all anatomic pathology services performed in 2010 across the three provider specialties—dermatology, gastroenterology, and urology—we reviewed. We then calculated the number of and expenditures for anatomic pathology services if self-referring providers performed biopsy procedures at the same rate as and referred the same number of services per biopsy procedure as non-self-referring providers of the same provider size and specialty. We repeated this analysis incorporating an approximation of the payment reduction for anatomic pathology services that became effective in 2013.[12]

We took several steps to ensure that the data used to produce this report were sufficiently reliable. Specifically, we assessed the reliability of the data we used from the Centers for Medicare & Medicaid Services (CMS)—the agency that administers Medicare—by interviewing officials responsible for overseeing these data sources, reviewing relevant documentation, and examining the data for obvious errors. We determined that the data were sufficiently reliable for the purposes of our study. For further information on the scope and methodology for this report, see appendix II.

We conducted this performance audit from January 2012 through June 2013 in accordance with generally accepted government auditing standards. Those standards require that we plan and perform the audit to obtain sufficient, appropriate evidence to provide a reasonable basis for our findings and conclusions based on our audit objectives. We believe that the evidence obtained provides a reasonable basis for our findings and conclusions based on our audit objectives.

BACKGROUND

Anatomic pathology services aid in the diagnosis and treatment of diseases such as cancers and gastroenteritis—a condition that causes irritation and inflammation of the stomach and intestines. Medicare pays providers for performing the services and subsequently interpreting the results. Payment for the performance of the services can be made through different payment systems, depending on where the anatomic pathology service is performed.

In 2010, Medicare paid about $1.28 billion under the physician fee schedule for anatomic pathology services across all settings, of which about $945 million was for services performed in physician offices and independent laboratories.

Anatomic Pathology Services

Anatomic pathology services involve the examination of tissues and other specimens to diagnose diseases, such as cancers and gastroenteritis, and guide patient care. The services may be performed after a biopsy procedure used to obtain tissue samples. For example, after removing tissue samples during a biopsy procedure on a patient's prostate, a urologist may refer the patient's tissue sample for examination to determine whether, on the basis of an analysis of the tissue sample or samples, the patient has prostate cancer. After collecting these tissue samples, a non-self-referring provider may send them to an independent diagnostic laboratory, a hospital laboratory, or pathology physician group for further preparation and analysis. In contrast, self-referring providers may prepare specimens or evaluate specimens or both at their practices, rather than involving an external diagnostic laboratory or pathology physician group. For example, the ordering provider's group practice may have a technician who prepares specimens into slides or include a pathologist who interprets these specimens, or both.

Providers have discretion in determining the number and type of tissue samples that become a specimen. For example, a provider referring anatomic pathology services may include more than one tissue sample in a specimen if the samples are from the same areas of abnormal tissue (see figure 1). Alternatively, a provider may choose to create multiple specimens, each containing a single tissue sample. Providers differ on whether or to what extent tissue samples can be combined in creating a specimen or if each tissue sample must become a specimen. For example, urologists differ on whether it is clinically appropriate to combine tissue samples obtained through a prostate biopsy procedure or whether each tissue sample must became a specimen. The resultant number of specimens has implications for payment as each specimen submitted for analysis can be billed to Medicare separately as an anatomic pathology service. CMS policy states that specimens submitted for individual examination should be medically reasonable and necessary for diagnosis. Finally, a pathologist—a specialty provider trained to interpret specimens—examines the specimen with and without a microscope and prepares written results of this examination for the referring provider.

Depending on the level of complexity, biopsy procedures can involve risks for patients. For example, biopsies of the skin to detect cancer are generally considered safe, but complications such as bleeding, bruising, or infection can occur.[13] Additional complications, such as difficulty urinating and infections resulting in hospitalization, can occur from other biopsy procedures.

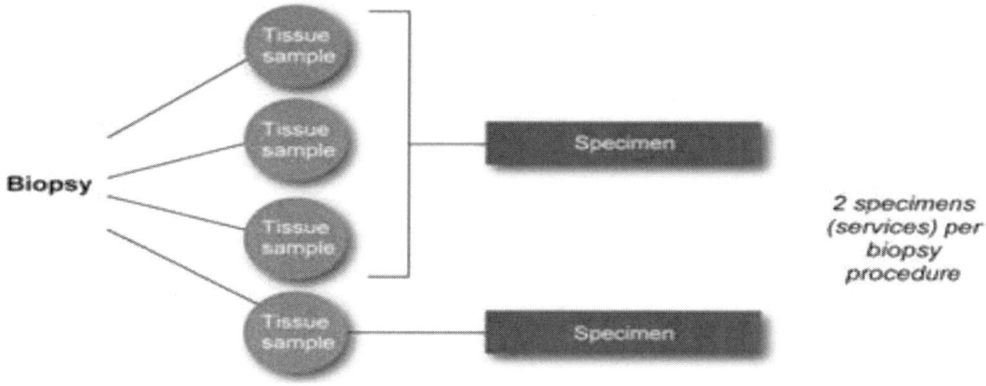

Source: GAO.

Note: Two specimens—anatomic pathology services—are prepared from four tissue samples in figure 1. Providers have the discretion to determine the number of samples that become specimens, so alternatively, four specimens could have been prepared from these four tissue samples. The resultant number of specimens has implications for payment as each specimen submitted for analysis can be billed to Medicare separately as an anatomic pathology service.

Figure 1. Preparation of Specimens from Tissue Samples.

Medicare Payment and Billing Policies for Anatomic Pathology Services

Medicare's payments for anatomic pathology services are separated into two components—the technical component (TC) and the professional component (PC). The TC payment is intended to cover the cost of preparing a specimen for analysis, including the costs for equipment, supplies, and nonphysician staff. The PC payment is intended to cover the provider's time examining the specimen and writing a report on the findings. The PC and TC can be billed together, on what is called a global claim, or alternatively the components can be billed separately. For instance, a global claim could be billed if the same provider prepares and examines the specimen, whereas the TC and PC could be billed separately if the performing and interpreting providers are different.

Medicare reimburses providers through different payment systems depending on where the anatomic pathology service is performed. When an anatomic pathology service is performed in a provider's office or independent clinical laboratory, both the PC and TC are reimbursed under the Medicare physician fee schedule. Alternatively when the service is performed in an institutional setting such as a hospital inpatient department, the provider is reimbursed under the Medicare physician fee schedule for the PC, while the TC is reimbursed under a different Medicare payment system. For instance, the TC of an anatomic pathology service performed in a hospital inpatient setting is reimbursed through a facility payment made under Medicare Part A.

Certain Policies Implemented by CMS Regarding Anatomic Pathology Services

In response to concerns about potential overutilization of anatomic pathology services due to physician self-referral, CMS established rules limiting the reimbursements allowed under certain self-referral arrangements. Specifically, in 2008 CMS imposed an "anti-markup rule" that prohibits providers from billing Medicare for anatomic pathology services for amounts that exceed what the providers themselves pay to subcontract the services from other providers or pathology laboratories.[14] However, in the 2009 physician fee schedule final rule, CMS identified an exception to the anti-markup rule: a service may be marked up when performed by a physician who shares a practice with the billing provider.[15] Since then, arrangements in which a provider group practice includes a pathologist in the practice's office space have become a common self-referral arrangement.

In the 2009 physician fee schedule, CMS also introduced a payment change for anatomic pathology services related to a specific biopsy procedure due to concern of overpayment. Specifically, CMS began paying for multiple anatomic pathology services from prostate saturation biopsy procedures through a single payment, rather than paying for each specimen individually. This specific biopsy procedure involves taking numerous tissue samples—typically 30 to 60—to increase the likelihood of detecting prostate cancer in a subgroup of high-risk individuals in whom previous conventional prostate biopsies had been negative. As a result, CMS introduced four new HCPCS codes to pay for these specimens, which were previously paid through HCPCS 88305.[16] The four HCPCS codes noted are payment for 1 to 20 specimens (G0416), 21 to 40 specimens (G0417), 41 to 60 specimens (G0418), and more than 60 specimens (G0419).[17] The payment change resulted in a substantial decrease in payment for anatomic pathology services resulting from prostate saturation biopsy procedures.[18]

CMS reduced its payment for anatomic pathology services in 2013 as part of its efforts to examine the payment for certain high-volume services. Specifically, CMS reduced its payment of anatomic pathology services in 2013 because it determined that fewer resources—equipment, supplies, and nonphysician staff—were required to prepare anatomic pathology services, which in turn reduced payment for the TC. Effective January 1, 2013, CMS reduced Medicare's reimbursement for anatomic pathology services under the physician fee schedule by lowering reimbursement for the TC by approximately half. With this change, a payment for a global claim for an anatomic pathology service was reduced by approximately 30 percent.[19]

2010 Anatomic Pathology Services Utilization and Expenditures

In 2010, there were about 16.2 million anatomic pathology services performed in all settings, including physician offices and hospitals. In 2010, expenditures for anatomic pathology services paid under the physician fee schedule totaled about $1.28 billion across all settings. About $945 million of the $1.28 billion—74 percent—in expenditures for anatomic pathology services in 2010 were for services performed in physician offices and independent laboratories.

SELF-REFERRED ANATOMIC PATHOLOGY SERVICES AND EXPENDITURES GREW FASTER THAN NON-SELF-REFERRED SERVICES AND EXPENDITURES

The number of self-referred anatomic pathology services increased at a faster rate than non-self-referred anatomic pathology services from 2004 through 2010. Similarly, expenditures for self-referred anatomic pathology services increased at a faster rate than expenditures for non-self-referred services. The share of anatomic pathology services that were self-referred increased overall during the period we reviewed.

Number of Self-referred Anatomic Pathology Services Increased at a Faster Rate Than Non-selfreferred Services

While both the number of self-referred and non-self-referred anatomic pathology services grew overall from 2004 through 2010, self-referred services increased at a faster rate than non-self-referred services. Specifically, the number of self-referred anatomic pathology services more than doubled over the period we reviewed, growing from about 1.06 million services in 2004 to about 2.26 million services in 2010 (see figure 2).[20] In contrast, the number of non-self-referred anatomic pathology services increased about 38 percent, growing from about 5.64 million services to about 7.77 million services. Because of the faster growth in self-referred anatomic pathology services, the proportion of anatomic pathology services that were self-referred grew from about 15.9 percent in 2004 to about 22.5 percent in 2010. Notably, the number of self-referred anatomic pathology services increased from 2004 through 2010, even after accounting for the decrease in the number of Medicare FFS beneficiaries.[21] Specifically, the number of self-referred anatomic pathology services per 1,000 Medicare FFS beneficiaries grew from about 30 to about 64, an increase of about 113 percent. Although both self-referred and non-self-referred anatomic pathology services increased over the period of our study, the number of self-referred anatomic pathology services decreased slightly from about 1.67 million in 2007 to about 1.65 million in 2008 before increasing about 14 percent to 1.88 million services in 2009.[22] This decrease in 2008 corresponds to the implementation of CMS's anti-markup rule that limits reimbursement for anatomic pathology services in certain self-referral arrangements. In contrast, the number of non-self-referred anatomic pathology services increased every year during the period we studied, with the largest annual increase (about 13 percent) in 2008.

Medicare's Expenditures for Self-referred Anatomic Pathology Services Grew Faster Than Expenditures for Non-self-referred Services

While Medicare expenditures for self-referred and non-self-referred anatomic pathology services grew from 2004 through 2010, expenditures for the self-referred services increased at a faster rate. Specifically, expenditures for self-referred anatomic pathology services grew about 164 percent from 2004 to 2010, increasing from about $75 million in 2004 to $199 million in 2010 (see figure 3). In contrast, non-self-referred anatomic pathology expenditures increased about 57 percent, from $473 million to about $741 million.

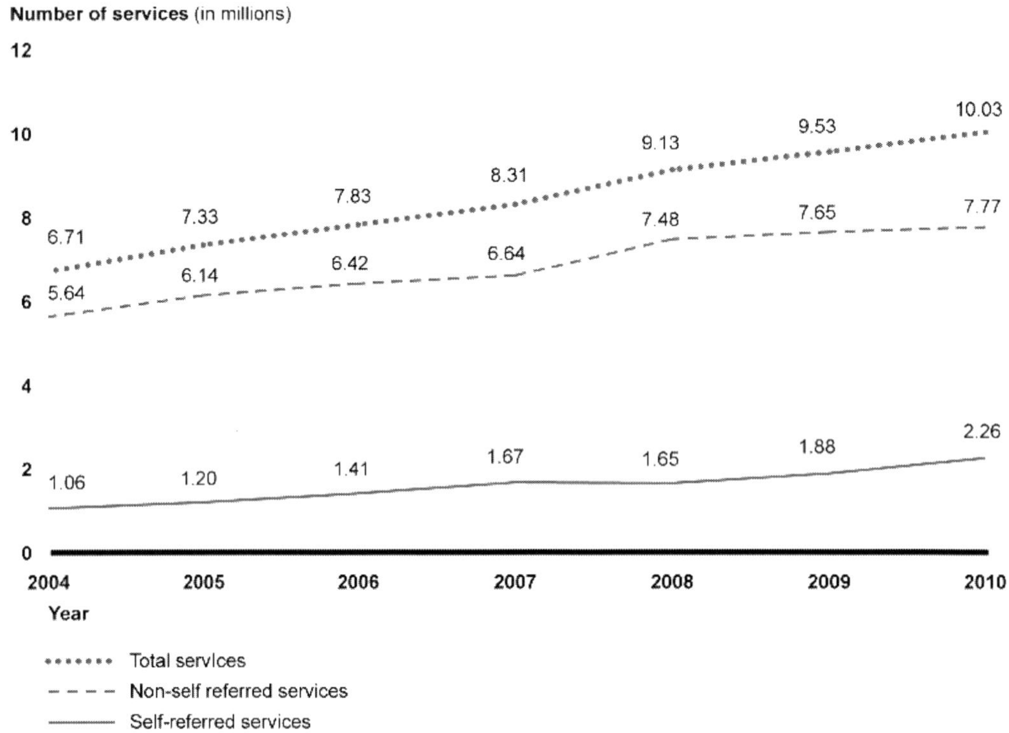

Source: GAO analysis of CMS data.

Note: Results include services performed in a physician's office or diagnostic laboratory for services with a Healthcare Common Procedure Coding System (HCPCS) code of 88305. Services performed in other settings, such as hospital outpatient departments, are not included.

Figure 2. Number of Self-referred and Non-self-referred Medicare Anatomic Pathology Services, 2004–2010.

Share of Self-referred Anatomic Pathology Services Increased across Provider Specialties Referring Most Anatomic Pathology Services

Consistent with the overall trend, the proportion of anatomic pathology services that were self-referred increased for the three provider specialties—dermatology, gastroenterology, and urology—that accounted for over 90 percent of self-referred anatomic pathology services in 2010 (see table 1). For example, the proportion of anatomic pathology services self-referred by dermatologists increased from 24 percent in 2004 to about 29 percent in 2010.

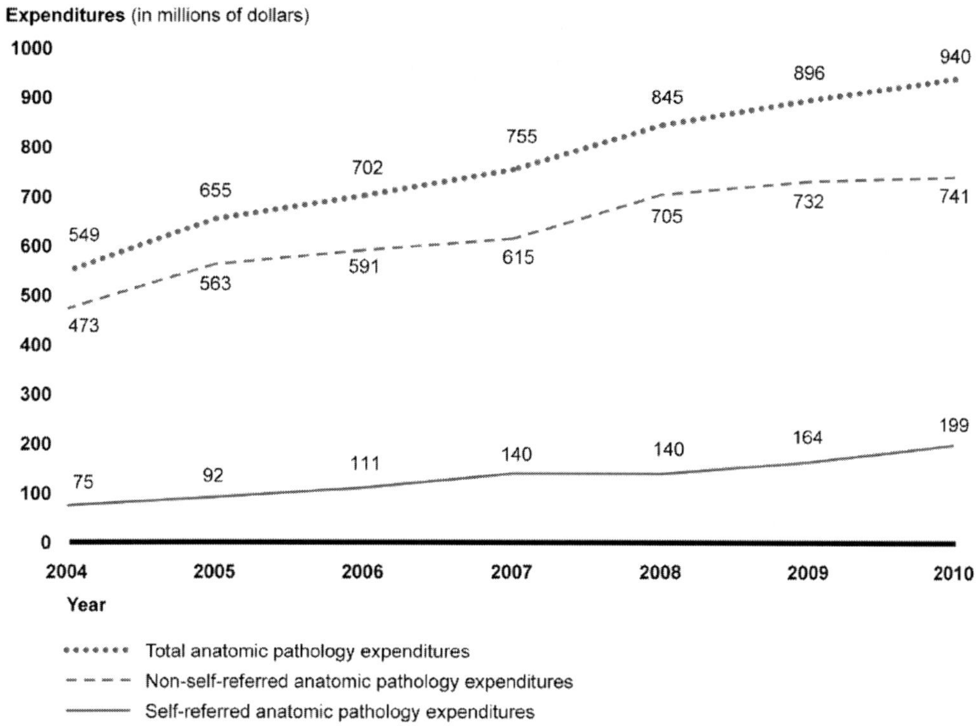

Source: GAO analysis of CMS data.

Note: Results include expenditures for anatomic pathology services performed in a physician's office or diagnostic laboratory for Healthcare Common Procedure Coding System (HCPCS) code 88305. Services performed in other settings, such as hospital outpatient departments, are not included.

Figure 3. Expenditures for Self-referred and Non-self-referred Medicare Anatomic Pathology Services, 2004–2010.

Table 1. Change in Self-referral Rates for Medicare Anatomic Pathology Services from 2004 to 2010 for Select Provider Specialties

Provider specialty	Percentage of anatomic pathology services self-referred in 2004	Percentage of anatomic pathology services self-referred in 2010	Percentage ofself-referredservices referred byspecialty in 2010
Dermatology	24.0%	29.3%	58.9%
Urology	13.9	32.5	16.4
Gastroenterology	6.6	20.9	14.9
Total	N/A	N/A	90.2%

Source: GAO analysis of CMS data.

Note: No other provider specialty referred more than 2 percent of self-referred anatomic pathology services in both 2004 and 2010.

SELF-REFERRING PROVIDERS GENERALLY REFERRED MORE ANATOMIC PATHOLOGY SERVICES ON AVERAGE THAN NON-SELF-REFERRING PROVIDERS

Self-referring providers in 2010 generally referred more anatomic pathology services on average than those providers who did not self-refer these services, even after accounting for differences in specialty, number of Medicare FFS beneficiaries seen, patient characteristics, or geography. Providers' referrals for anatomic pathology services substantially increased the year after they began to self-refer.

Self-referring Providers Generally Referred More Anatomic Pathology Services Than Other Providers Regardless of Practice or Patient Characteristics

Across the three provider specialties—dermatology, gastroenterology, and urology—that refer the majority of anatomic pathology services, we found that in 2010, self-referring providers referred more anatomic pathology services, on average, than other providers, regardless of number of Medicare FFS beneficiaries seen. Specifically, we found this pattern for dermatologists, gastroenterologists, and urologists treating small, medium, and large numbers of Medicare beneficiaries (see table 2). Notably, for all provider specialties, providers who treated a large number of Medicare FFS beneficiaries—more than 500—had the highest relative rate within each specialty.

Table 2. Average Number of Medicare Anatomic Pathology Services Referred by Self-referring and Non-self-referring Providers for Select Provider Specialties in 2010

	Average number of anatomic pathology services referred		
Provider specialty and number of unique Medicare FFS beneficiaries[a]	Self-referring providers	Non-self-referring providers	Relative rate of self-referring providers[b]
Dermatology			
1 to 250	169	143	1.18
251 to 500	541	451	1.20
>500	1,583	1,013	1.56
Gastroenterology			
1 to 250	171	140	1.22
251 to 500	417	350	1.19
>500	813	645	1.26
Urology			
1 to 250	100	75	1.33
251 to 500	248	174	1.43
>500	465	303	1.53

Source: GAO analysis of CMS data.

Notes: We use the term anatomic pathology services to refer specifically to those services with a Healthcare Common Procedure Coding System (HCPCS) code of 88305, the examination of specimens from tissue samples taken through biopsy procedures.

Provider specialties above represent 29,870 providers who referred about 64 percent of anatomic pathology services across all settings during 2010. Providers were considered to be self-referring if they self-referred anatomic pathology services for at least one biopsy procedure. Of the 29,870 providers represented above that referred at least one beneficiary for an anatomic pathology service in 2010, 7,177 were self-referring and 22,693 were non-self-referring. Of the 7,177 self-referring providers, 3,364 were dermatologists, 1,769 were gastroenterologists, and 2,044 were urologists. Of the non-self-referring providers, 6,656 were dermatologists, 9,566 were gastroenterologists, and 6,471 were urologists.

[a]The number of unique Medicare fee-for-service (FFS) beneficiaries refers to the number of unique beneficiaries that received at least one service from a provider.

[b]The relative rate of self-referring providers refers to the factor by which the average number of anatomic pathology services referred by self-referring providers is greater or less than the average number of anatomic pathology services referred by non-self-referring providers. For example, if the relative rate of self-referring providers is equal to 2, it would mean that, on average, self-referring providers referred twice as many anatomic pathology services as non-self-referring providers.

Self-referring providers generally referred more anatomic pathology services on average than non-self-referring providers due to referring more services—specimens to be examined—per biopsy procedures and, in certain cases, performing a greater number of biopsy procedures. Across the three specialties we reviewed, self-referring providers referred more services per biopsy procedure, on average, than non-self-referring providers, regardless of the number of Medicare FFS beneficiaries seen. Specifically, self-referring providers referred from 7 percent to 52 percent more services per biopsy procedure for the provider specialty and size category combinations we examined. Further, we observed a greater number of biopsy procedures performed by self-referring providers in certain cases. Specifically, self-referring dermatologists treating medium and large numbers of Medicare FFS beneficiaries performed about 8 and 38 percent more biopsy procedures on average, respectively, than nonself-referring dermatologists treating similar numbers of Medicare beneficiaries.[23] In the remaining provider specialty and size category combinations, the rate of biopsy procedures performed by self-referring providers was similar to that for non-self-referring providers.

The higher number of referrals for anatomic pathology services among self-referring providers relative to other providers of the same size and specialty cannot, in general, be explained by differences in patient diagnoses, patient health status, other patient characteristics, or geography.

Patient Diagnoses

Differences in referrals for anatomic pathology services between self-referring and non-self-referring providers of the same specialty treating a similar number of Medicare FFS beneficiaries could not be explained by differences in their patients' diagnoses. Generally, we found that the types and proportions of patient diagnoses were similar for self-referring and non-self-referring providers of the same specialty. However, we found that self-referring providers referred more anatomic pathology services per biopsy procedure for nearly all—53 of 54—primary diagnoses for which beneficiaries were referred for anatomic pathology services.[24] This pattern is particularly evident for those diagnoses that accounted for a large proportion of anatomic pathology services referred within each specialty (see table 3). For example, self-referring urology providers referred on average about 12.5 anatomic pathology services per biopsy procedure for diagnosis of elevated prostate specific antigen (790.93) while non-self-referring urology providers referred about 8.5 anatomic pathology services per biopsy procedure for this diagnosis. For further information on the average number of anatomic pathology services referred per biopsy procedure by beneficiary primary diagnosis, see appendix III.

Table 3. Average Number of Medicare Anatomic Pathology Services per Biopsy Procedure for Most Common Diagnoses Referred by Self-referring and Non-self-referring Providers, Select Provider Specialties in 2010

	Average number of anatomic pathology services per biopsy procedure		
Provider specialty and most common diagnoses, including International Classification of Diseases, Ninth Revision, Clinical Modification (ICD-9-CM) diagnostic code	**Self-referring providers**	**Non-self-referring providers**	**Percentage difference**
Dermatology			
Neoplasm of uncertain behavior of skin (238.2)	1.8	1.6	13%
Other malignant neoplasm of skin of other and unspecified parts of face (173.3)	1.6	1.4	14
Actinic keratosis (702.0)	1.7	1.5	13
Gastroenterology			
Benign neoplasm of colon (211.3)	2.2	1.9	16
Atrophic gastritis, without mention of hemorrhage (535.10)	2.2	1.9	16
Unspecified gastritis and gastroduodenitis, without mention of hemorrhage (535.50)	2.7	2.0	35
Urology			
Elevated prostate specific antigen (790.93)	12.5	8.5	47
Malignant neoplasm of prostate (185)	8.5	6.1	39
Malignant neoplasm of bladder, part unspecified (188.9)	1.8	1.7	6

Source: GAO analysis of CMS data.

Note: Proportion of all diagnoses referred for anatomic pathology services represented by the three most common codes varies by specialty. Specifically, the three most common diagnoses account for 36.3 percent and 30.2 percent of biopsy procedures performed by self-referring and non-self-referring dermatologists, 43.2 percent and 44.7 percent of biopsy procedures performed by self-referring and non-self-referring gastroenterologists, and 50.3 percent and 46.6 percent of biopsy procedures performed by self-referring and non-self-referring urologists, respectively.

Patient Health Status

Differences in the number of referrals for anatomic pathology services between self-referring and non-self-referring providers of the same specialty treating similar numbers of Medicare FFS beneficiaries could generally not be explained by differences in patient health status. Specifically, for all three provider specialties we reviewed, the beneficiaries seen by self-referring providers treating a small, medium, or large number of Medicare FFS beneficiaries were of similar health status as patients seen by non-self-referring providers of the same specialty and size category (see table 4), as indicated by having similar average risk scores.[25] If self-referring providers saw relatively sicker beneficiaries, it could have explained why these providers referred more anatomic pathology services on average than other providers of the same provider specialty and size categories.

Table 4. Average Health Status of Medicare Beneficiaries for Select Provider Specialties by Practice Size in 2010

Provider specialty and number of unique Medicare fee-for-service (FFS) beneficiaries[a]	Average risk score of beneficiaries[b]	
	Self-referring providers	Non-self-referring providers
Dermatology		
1 to 250	1.20	1.18
251 to 500	1.15	1.15
> 500	1.12	1.13
Gastroenterology		
1 to 250	1.40	1.49
251 to 500	1.36	1.40
> 500	1.34	1.38
Urology		
1 to 250	1.37	1.40
251 to 500	1.37	1.36
> 500	1.35	1.33

Source: GAO analysis of CMS data.

[a]The number of unique Medicare FFS beneficiaries refers to the number of unique beneficiaries that received at least one service from a provider.

[b]A beneficiary's risk score is a proxy for health status and is equivalent to the ratio of expected health care expenditures for that beneficiary under Medicare FFS relative to the average health care expenditures for all Medicare FFS beneficiaries. For example, a beneficiary with a risk score of 1.05 would have expected expenditures that were 5 percent higher than an average Medicare FFS beneficiary. The risk scores presented are normalized using the FFS normalization factor of 1.041 that CMS used to normalize risk scores in 2010. Normalization keeps the average Medicare FFS risk score constant at 1.0 over time.

Other Patient Characteristics

Differences in the number of anatomic pathology service referrals between self-referring and non-self-referring providers of the same specialty treating similar numbers of Medicare FFS beneficiaries could not be explained by differences in the age and sex of beneficiaries. In particular, the age and sex of Medicare FFS beneficiaries were generally consistent between those beneficiaries seen by self-referring providers and those seen by non-self-referring providers for all provider specialties and size categories we examined. For further information on the average age and sex of beneficiaries seen by self-referring and non-self-referring providers of the provider specialties we examined, see appendix IV.

Geography

Differences in the number of anatomic pathology service referrals between self-referring and non-self-referring providers could not generally be explained by whether a provider practiced in an urban or rural area.

Self-referring providers of the same specialty treating a similar number of Medicare beneficiaries generally referred more anatomic pathology services on average than non-self-referring providers, regardless of whether the provider practiced in an urban or rural area. For example, self-referring dermatologists and urologists treating a similar number of Medicare FFS beneficiaries had higher referral rates on average for anatomic pathology services, regardless of whether they practiced in an urban or rural location. Likewise, self-referring gastroenterologists treating a medium or large number of Medicare FFS beneficiaries referred a higher number of anatomic pathology services on average than non-selfreferring gastroenterologists treating a similar number of Medicare beneficiaries, regardless of whether they practiced in an urban or rural location. For further information on referral of anatomic pathology services across provider specialties and size categories in urban and rural areas, see appendix V.

Providers' Referrals for Anatomic Pathology Services Increased the Year after They Began to Self-refer

Our analysis shows that, across the three provider specialties we reviewed, providers' referrals for anatomic pathology services substantially increased the year after they began to self-refer. In our analysis we examined the number of anatomic pathology referrals made by "switchers"—those providers that did not self-refer in 2007 or 2008 but began to self-refer in 2009 and continued to do so in 2010—and compared these referrals to the number made by providers that did not begin to self-refer during this period. Providers could self-refer by setting up an in-office laboratory, contracting for laboratory services, or joining a group practice that already self-referred. We found that the switchers saw large increases in the number of anatomic referrals they made from 2008 to 2010 when compared with other providers (see table 5). Specifically, across the three provider specialties we reviewed, the switcher group of providers increased the number of anatomic pathology referrals they made from 2008 to 2010 by at least 14.0 percent and by as much as 58.5 percent. In contrast, providers that self-referred anatomic pathology services during the entire period experienced smaller changes in the number of referrals, ranging from a 1.4 percent increase to an 11.6 percent increase, depending on the provider specialty. Among providers that did not self-refer anatomic pathology services, the number of referrals the providers made for these services ranged from a decrease of 0.2 percent to an increase of 2.8 percent, depending on the provider specialty.

Providers in the switcher groups for the three specialties we reviewed had an increase in the number of anatomic pathology referrals they made from 2008 to 2010 due to an increase, on average, in the number of anatomic pathology services referred per biopsy procedure. Across the three specialties we reviewed, the increase in the number of specimens submitted for examination from each biopsy procedure from 2008 to 2010 ranged from 13.3 percent to 48.9 percent. For all three specialties we reviewed, the increase in the number of anatomic pathology services referred per biopsy procedure was greater for providers in the switchers group than for providers who did not self-refer from 2008 through 2010 or those providers who self-referred for all 3 years.

Table 5. Change in Average Number of Medicare Anatomic Pathology Services Referred by Provider Specialty, 2008 and 2010

Primary specialty	Referral type	Number of providers	Average number of unique Medicare fee-for-service (FFS) beneficiaries, 2010	Anatomic pathology services, 2008[a]	Anatomic pathology services, 2010[a]	Percentage change 2008 to 2010
Dermatology	Switchers	130	478.2	658.6	815.5	23.8%
	Self-referring	1,353	573.6	803.9	815.0	1.4
	Non-self-referring	2,361	424.4	451.9	453.2	0.3
Gastroenterology	Switchers	195	335.5	338.7	386.1	14.0
	Self-referring	438	380.9	413.7	439.6	6.3
	Non-self-referring	4,833	365.1	340.8	350.4	2.8
Urology	Switchers	215	619.1	257.3	407.7	58.5
	Self-referring	498	626.8	289.4	322.9	11.6
	Non-self-referring	3,192	473.6	175.8	175.4	-0.2

Source: GAO analysis of CMS data.

Notes: Anatomic pathology services refer specifically to services with Healthcare Common Procedure Coding System (HCPCS) code 88305. We define switchers as those providers that did not self-refer in 2007 or 2008, but did self-refer in 2009 and 2010.

[a]The average number of anatomic pathology services referred by self-referring providers, non-selfreferring providers, and switchers are influenced in part by the average number of unique Medicare FFS beneficiaries seen by each referral type. For example, in 2008, both switchers—who did not self-refer in 2008—and non-self-referring urologists averaged approximately 0.4 anatomic pathology referrals per unique Medicare FFS beneficiary. However, switchers averaged more anatomic pathology referrals than non-self-referring providers in 2008 because they saw, on average, more unique Medicare FFS beneficiaries.

The increase in anatomic pathology referrals for providers that began self-referring in 2009 cannot be explained exclusively by factors such as providers joining practices with higher patient volumes, different patient populations, or different practice cultures. Specifically, providers that remained in the same practice from 2007 through 2010, but began self-referring in 2009, also had a bigger increase in the number of anatomic pathology referrals than did providers that did not change their self-referral status. The increase in the number of anatomic pathology services referred by providers in the switcher group that met this criterion from 2008 to 2010 ranged from an increase of 6.8 percent to an increase of 38.6 percent, depending on the provider specialty.

HIGHER USE OF ANATOMIC PATHOLOGY SERVICES BY SELF-REFERRING PROVIDERS RESULTS IN SUBSTANTIAL ADDITIONAL MEDICARE SPENDING

We estimate that Medicare spent about $69 million more in 2010 than the program would have spent if self-referring providers performed biopsy procedures at the same rate as and referred the same number of services per biopsy procedure as non-self-referring providers of the same provider size and specialty (see figure 4).[26]

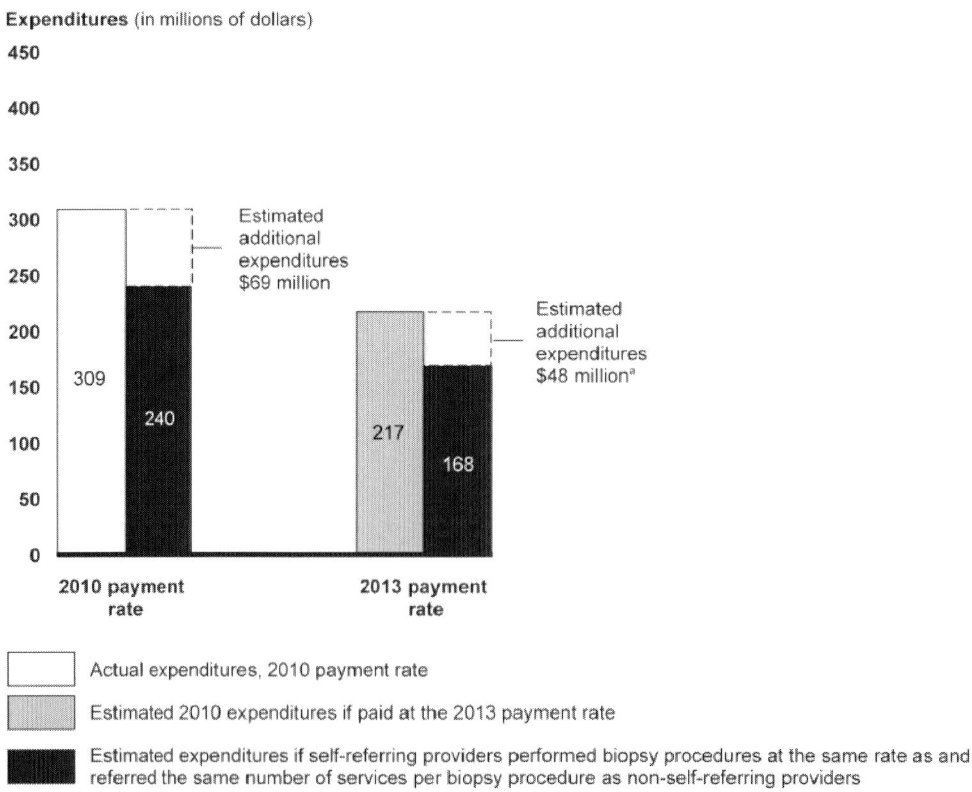

Source: GAO analysis of CMS data.

Notes: Anatomic pathology services refer specifically to services with Healthcare Common Procedure Coding System (HCPCS) code 88305. Our analysis included expenditures for anatomic pathology services referred by dermatologists, gastroenterologists, and urologists. Combined, these three specialties were responsible for approximately 64 percent of all referrals for anatomic pathology services and 90 percent of all self-referred anatomic pathology services in 2010. We calculated expenditures for services as if self-referring providers performed biopsy procedures at the same rate as and referred the same number of services per biopsy procedure as non-self-referring providers of the same specialty and size in 2010. To estimate expenditures for 2010 as though the 2013 payment rate were in effect, we reduced expenditures for anatomic pathology services by 30 percent.

These 2013 estimated expenditures do not include the payment reductions that may result from implementation of the Budget Control Act of 2011, Pub. L. No. 112-25, 125 Stat. 240, as amended by the American Taxpayer Relief Act of 2012 (Pub. L. No. 112-240, 126 Stat. 2313) (2013).

[a]Estimated additional expenditures at the 2013 payment rate do not equal the difference of estimated 2010 expenditures if paid at the 2013 payment rate and the estimated expenditures if self-referring providers performed biopsy procedures at the same rate as and referred the same number of services per biopsy procedure as non-self-referring providers due to rounding.

Figure 4. Estimated Additional Medicare Spending for Anatomic Pathology Services Attributed to Self-Referring Providers, 2010.

This additional spending can be attributed to the fact that self-referring providers in the 3 provider specialties we examined referred about 918,000 more anatomic pathology services in 2010. In 2013, CMS reduced its payment of anatomic pathology services because it determined that fewer resources—equipment, supplies, and non-physician staff—were required to prepare anatomic pathology services. If the lower 2013 Medicare reimbursement rates for anatomic pathology services were in effect in 2010, Medicare would have spent approximately $48 million more than it would have if self-referring providers performed biopsy procedures at the same rate as and referred the same number of services per biopsy procedure as non-self-referring providers of the same provider size and specialty.

This calculation likely underestimates the total amount of additional Medicare spending that can be attributed to self-referring providers because we did not include all Medicare providers in our analysis. Specifically, we limited our analysis to anatomic pathology services referred by dermatologists, gastroenterologists, and urologists. These specialties account for approximately 64 percent of anatomic pathology services referred across all settings and about 90 percent of all self-referred anatomic pathology services in 2010.

CONCLUSION

Anatomic pathology services are vital services that help providers diagnose disease and guide treatment options for patient care. Proponents of self-referral contend that the ability of providers to self-refer anatomic pathology services has the potential benefit of more rapid diagnoses and better coordination of care. Our review indicates that across the major provider specialties that refer beneficiaries for anatomic pathology services, self-referring providers generally referred more anatomic pathology services on average than other providers of the same specialty treating similar numbers of Medicare patients. This increase is due to a greater number of specimens submitted for examination from each biopsy procedure, and in certain cases a greater number of biopsy procedures performed. This increase raises concerns, in part because biopsy procedures, although generally safe, can result in serious complications for Medicare beneficiaries. Further, our analysis shows that across these provider specialties, providers' referrals for anatomic pathology services substantially increased the year after they began to self-refer.

The relatively higher rate of anatomic pathology services among self-referring providers cannot be explained by patient diagnosis, patient health status, or geographic location. Taken together, this suggests that financial incentives for self-referring providers were likely a major factor driving the increase in anatomic pathology referrals. In 2010, providers who self-referred made an estimated 918,000 more referrals for anatomic pathology services than they likely would have if they were not self-referring. Notably, these additional referrals cost CMS about $69 million in 2010 alone. To the extent that these additional services are unnecessary, avoiding them could result in savings to Medicare and to beneficiaries.

Despite the potential safety and financial implications of unnecessary anatomic pathology services, CMS does not have policies to address the effect of how self-referral affects the utilization of and expenditures for anatomic pathology services. CMS does not currently have the ability to identify anatomic pathology services that are self-referred so that the agency can track the extent to which anatomic pathology services are self-referred and identify services that may be unnecessary. Specifically, Medicare claims do not include an indicator or "flag" that identifies whether services are self-referred or non-self-referred. Thus, CMS does not currently have a method for easily identifying such services and cannot determine the effect of self-referral on utilization and expenditures for anatomic pathology services. Including a self-referral flag on Medicare Part B claims submitted by providers who bill for anatomic pathology services is likely the easiest and most cost-effective approach.

If CMS could readily identify self-referred anatomic pathology services, the agency may be better positioned to identify potentially inappropriate utilization of biopsy procedures. CMS could, for example, consider performing targeted audits of providers who perform a higher average number of biopsy procedures, compared to providers of the same specialty treating a similar number of Medicare beneficiaries. Given our report findings, CMS may want to initially focus its efforts on self-referring dermatologists who treated a larger number of Medicare beneficiaries.

While providers have discretion in determining the number of tissue samples that become specimens, CMS's current payment system provides a financial incentive for providers to refer a higher number of specimens—or anatomic pathology services—per biopsy procedure. Providers can double their payment for anatomic pathology services, for example, by submitting four specimens from four tissue samples instead of combining the four tissue samples into two specimens. However, providers differ on whether or to what extent tissue samples can be combined in creating a specimen or if each tissue sample must become a specimen. CMS has already implemented a payment approach for one specific biopsy procedure—prostate saturation biopsy—that pays providers through a single payment rather than paying for each specimen individually within a given range of anatomic pathology services, such as 1 to 20 specimens. However, this policy does not apply to anatomic pathology services from other biopsy procedures. CMS could expand this payment approach to other biopsy procedures and associated anatomic pathology services.

RECOMMENDATIONS FOR EXECUTIVE ACTION

In order to improve CMS's ability to identify self-referred anatomic pathology services and help CMS avoid unnecessary increases in these services, we recommend that the Administrator of CMS take the following three actions:

1) Insert a self-referral flag on Medicare Part B claim forms and require providers to indicate whether the anatomic pathology services for which the provider bills Medicare are self-referred or not.
2) Determine and implement an approach to ensure the appropriateness of biopsy procedures performed by self-referring providers.
3) Develop and implement a payment approach for anatomic pathology services that would limit the financial incentives associated with referring a higher number of specimens—or anatomic pathology services—per biopsy procedure.

AGENCY AND THIRD-PARTY COMMENTS AND OUR EVALUATION

We provided a draft of this report to HHS, which oversees CMS, for comment. HHS provided written comments. We also obtained comments from representatives from four professional associations selected because they represent an array of stakeholders with specific involvement in anatomic pathology services. Three associations provided oral comments: the College of American Pathologists (CAP), which represents pathologists; the American Academy of Dermatology Association (AADA), which represents dermatologists; and the American Gastroenterological Association (AGA), which represents gastroenterologists. The American Urological Association (AUA), which represents urologists, provided written comments. We summarize and respond to comments from HHS and representatives from the four professional associations in the following sections.

HHS Comments

In its comments, HHS stated that it concurred with, and had addressed, one of our recommendations, but did not concur with our other two recommendations. HHS provided few comments on our findings that self-referring providers referred substantially more anatomic pathology services than non-self-referring providers.

HHS stated that it concurred with, and has already addressed, our recommendation that CMS develop and implement a payment approach for anatomic pathology services that would limit the financial incentives associated with referring a higher number of anatomic pathology services per biopsy procedure. According to HHS, the payment revaluation for anatomic pathology services in 2013 decreased payment by approximately 30 percent and significantly reduced the financial incentives associated with self-referral for these services. We are pleased that CMS examines and revalues HCPCS codes to ensure that payment for services matches the resources involved and adjusts payment to the extent needed. However, the payment revaluation that occurred in 2013 does not address the higher referral of anatomic pathology services we found associated with self-referring providers. Although no consensus exists on the number and type of tissue samples that become a specimen—an anatomic pathology service—the current payment system pays more if providers create more specimens from the same number of samples. We continue to believe that CMS should develop a payment approach that addresses the incentive to provide more services.

HHS did not concur with our recommendation that CMS insert a self-referral flag on the Medicare Part B claims form and require providers to indicate whether the anatomic pathology services for which a provider bills Medicare are self-referred or not. In its response, HHS did not provide reasons for not concurring with this recommendation, but stated that the President's fiscal year 2014 budget proposal includes a provision to exclude certain services from the in-office ancillary services exception. HHS added that anatomic pathology services may share some characteristics with the services mentioned in the proposal. To the extent that self-referral for anatomic pathology services continues to be permitted, we believe that including an indicator or flag on the claims would likely be the easiest and most cost-effective approach to improve CMS's ability to identify self-referred anatomic pathology services. Such a flag would allow CMS to monitor the behavior of self-referring providers and could be helpful to CMS in answering broader policy questions on self-referral.

HHS did not concur with our recommendation that CMS determine and implement an approach to ensure the appropriateness of biopsy procedures performed by self-referring providers. In its response, HHS noted that it would be difficult to make recommendations regarding whether services are appropriate without reviewing large numbers of claims, reporting that 918,000 instances of self-referral that we identified would need to be reviewed. Further, the agency stated that it does not believe that this recommendation will address overutilization that occurs as a result of self-referral. We do not suggest or intend that CMS review every anatomic pathology service to determine whether it is appropriate. Self-referral, however, could be a factor CMS considers in its ongoing efforts to identify and address inappropriate use of Medicare services. As noted in the report, CMS could, for example, consider performing targeted audits of providers that perform a higher average number of biopsy procedures, compared to providers of the same specialty treating similar numbers of Medicare beneficiaries. In this regard, a flag that we also recommended to identify self-referred services would facilitate such audits.

On the basis of HHS's written response to our report, we are concerned that HHS does not appear to recognize the need to monitor the self-referral of anatomic pathology services on an ongoing basis and determine those services that may be inappropriate or unnecessary. HHS did not comment on our key finding that providers' referrals for anatomic pathology services across the three specialties we examined substantially increased the year after they began to self-refer. Nor did HHS comment on our estimate that additional referrals for anatomic pathology services from self-referring providers cost CMS about $69 million in 2010 or $48 million based on the 2013 payment rates. Given these findings, we continue to believe that CMS should take steps to monitor the utilization of anatomic pathology services and ensure that the services for which Medicare pays are appropriate. By not monitoring the appropriateness of these services, CMS is missing an opportunity to save Medicare expenditures.

Professional Association Comments College of American Pathologists

Representatives from CAP expressed concern that our methodology to identify self-referral missed certain self-referral arrangements for anatomic pathology services and that our findings understate effects from self-referral. According to the CAP representatives, because our methodology did not identify providers who self-refer the PC only and did not include financial relationships that do not share TINs, effects from self-referral are greater than our findings suggest. As noted in the report, we excluded claims with a only a PC from our finding on utilization and expenditures trends for anatomic pathology services because we could not reliably determine that they were performed in the physician office or independent laboratory. We identified financial relationships among providers using TINs, which would identify the provider, the provider's employer, or another entity to which the provider reassigns payment. To the extent that providers self-refer only the PCs of anatomic pathology services or self-refer to entities with which they do not share TINs, differences between self-referring and non-self-referring providers would be greater, and our estimate of the differences would be more conservative. CAP representatives also raised questions about self-referral that our report did not address, such as why the report did not examine cancer detection rates or whether anatomic pathology services should be included in the in-office ancillary services exception. These issues were outside the report's objectives. While the representatives from CAP agreed with the recommendation to include a self-referral flag on the Medicare Part B claims form, they disagreed with our other recommendations, stating that they would not sufficiently address the report findings. We believe that our recommendations incorporate actions that address the problems we identified.

American Academy of Dermatology Association

Representatives from the AADA stated that dermatologists should continue to be allowed to prepare and review their own anatomic pathology services because they receive considerable training as part of their education and offered several possible explanations for the additional anatomic pathology services referred and biopsy procedures performed by self-referring providers. For example, they raised the possibility that the increase in anatomic pathology services referred and biopsy procedures performed by providers in the switcher group was due to increases in patient volume, providers joining a larger group practice or hiring a mid-level practitioner allowing the provider to see more patients. They also raised the possibility that providers in the switcher group became further specialized, resulting in a change in the number and type of diagnoses for their patients. Also, the AADA reported that our reliance on TINs to identify self-referral could be problematic because providers working in large, university-based practices would be flagged as self-referring, despite lacking a financial incentive to provide more services. As noted in the report, the increase in anatomic pathology referrals for providers that began self-referring in 2009 cannot be explained exclusively by factors such as providers joining practices with higher patient volumes, different patient populations, or different practice cultures. Specifically, providers that remained in the same practice from 2007 through 2010, but began self-referring in 2009, had a bigger increase in the number of anatomic pathology services referred than providers who did not change their self-referral status. Further, we found that the types and proportions of patient diagnoses were similar for self-referring and non-self-referring providers of the same specialty and that self-referring providers referred more anatomic pathology services per biopsy procedure for nearly all—53 of 54—primary diagnoses for which beneficiaries were referred for anatomic pathology services. To the extent that providers who share a TIN, but do not have a financial incentive to refer more services, are counted as self-referring, our findings would likely underestimate differences between self-referring and non-selfreferring providers and would thus provide a conservative estimate of the effects of self-referral.

The AADA agreed with our recommendation of determining an approach to ensure the appropriateness of biopsy procedures, but disagreed with our recommendation of a payment approach limiting the financial incentives associated with a higher number of services per biopsy procedure. Specifically, the AADA expressed concern about any disincentives for dermatologists to perform biopsy procedures. As noted in the report, increases in the number of anatomic pathology services per biopsy procedure were primarily responsible for the growth of anatomic pathology services referred by providers in the switcher group from 2008 to 2010 across provider specialties. We continue to believe that CMS should develop and implement a payment approach for anatomic pathology services that would limit the financial incentives associated with referring a higher number of services per biopsy procedure.

American Gastroenterological Association

Representatives from the AGA asked for further information about the providers in our analysis (particularly gastroenterologists in the switcher group) and diagnoses of the beneficiaries referred for anatomic pathology services, and offered several possible explanations for the additional anatomic pathology services referred and biopsy procedures performed by self-referring providers. Specifically, the AGA raised the possibility that providers in the switcher group joined larger groups that perform more anatomic pathology services or changed the types of biopsy procedures they performed. Finally, the AGA also noted that an appropriate number of anatomic pathology services is not known. Specifically, they reported that larger practices, which are also more likely to self-refer, are more likely to have formal peer review, which could result in more anatomic pathology services referred. We have included an appendix with additional information on the number of services per biopsy procedure for the most common diagnoses for which beneficiaries were referred for anatomic pathology services in 2010. As noted, the types and proportions of diagnoses for which beneficiaries were referred for anatomic pathology services were similar for self-referring and non-self-referring providers. We found that self-referring providers referred more services per biopsy procedure on average than non-self-referring providers for nearly all of these diagnoses. We acknowledge that the appropriate number of referrals for these services is not known, but the consistent pattern of self-referring providers' higher use suggests that additional scrutiny is warranted. The AGA agreed with our recommendations, but did not think the recommendation on a payment approach for anatomic pathology services limiting the financial incentives associated with referring a higher number of specimens per biopsy procedure was as applicable to providers of their specialty.

American Urological Association

The AUA agreed with our recommendation to identify self-referred services but did not agree with our other recommendations to examine the appropriateness of biopsy procedures performed by self-referring providers or develop a payment approach that would limit the financial incentives for referring a higher number of anatomic pathology services. The AUA said that there were problems with the study's design and data gathering methodology originating from problems with identifying self-referral which resulted in their questioning the validity of the report findings. AUA did not provide further detail on their methodological concerns. We believe our methodology to identify self-referred services and classify providers as self-referring using one hundred percent of Medicare Part B claims is a reasonable and valid approach. In designing our methodology, we consulted with officials from CMS, specialty societies, and other researchers. Our approach is similar to the one used by MedPAC for its study of the effect of physician self-referral on use of imaging services.[27]

James C. Cosgrove
Director, Health Care

APPENDIX I: SPECIAL STAINS USED IN CONJUNCTION WITH ANATOMIC PATHOLOGY SERVICES PAID UNDER MEDICARE

As part of our work, we also analyzed additional anatomic pathology services—known as special stains—that providers may use in conjunction with anatomic pathology services to enhance their ability in making a diagnosis. We focused our special stains analysis on services with Healthcare Common Procedure Coding System (HCPCS) codes 88312, 88313, and 88342 that were used in conjunction with the anatomic pathology service, HCPCS code 88305.

We considered special stains billed on the same date, by the same provider, for the same beneficiary as those used in conjunction with anatomic pathology services. In 2010, expenditures under the physician fee schedule for these three special stain services totaled approximately $387 million.

Providers may utilize special stains with a HCPCS code of 88312 on specimens to detect the presence of infectious organisms such as bacteria and fungus, special stains with a HCPCS code of 88313 to detect the presence of iron, and special stains with a HCPCS code of 88342 to identify the origin of a cancer.[1] Use of special stains is determined by the provider referring anatomic pathology services, the pathologist interpreting the anatomic pathology service, or both.

We examined (1) trends in the number of and expenditures for self-referred and non-self-referred special stains, and (2) how the provision of special stains differs for providers who self-refer when compared with other providers.

Utilization of and Expenditures for Self-Referred and Non-Self-Referred Special Stains

Similar to anatomic pathology services, the number of both self-referred and non-self-referred special stains increased from 2004 through 2010, with self-referred special stains increasing at a faster rate than services that were not self-referred. Specifically, the number of special stains that were self-referred increased from about 60,000 in 2004 to about 340,000 in 2010, an increase of more than 400 percent (see figure 5). Further, we found that self-referred special stains increased more than non-selfreferred special stains for each of the three special stains we studied. In contrast, non-self-referred special stains grew from about 710,000 services to about 1.80 million services, an increase of about 150 percent.

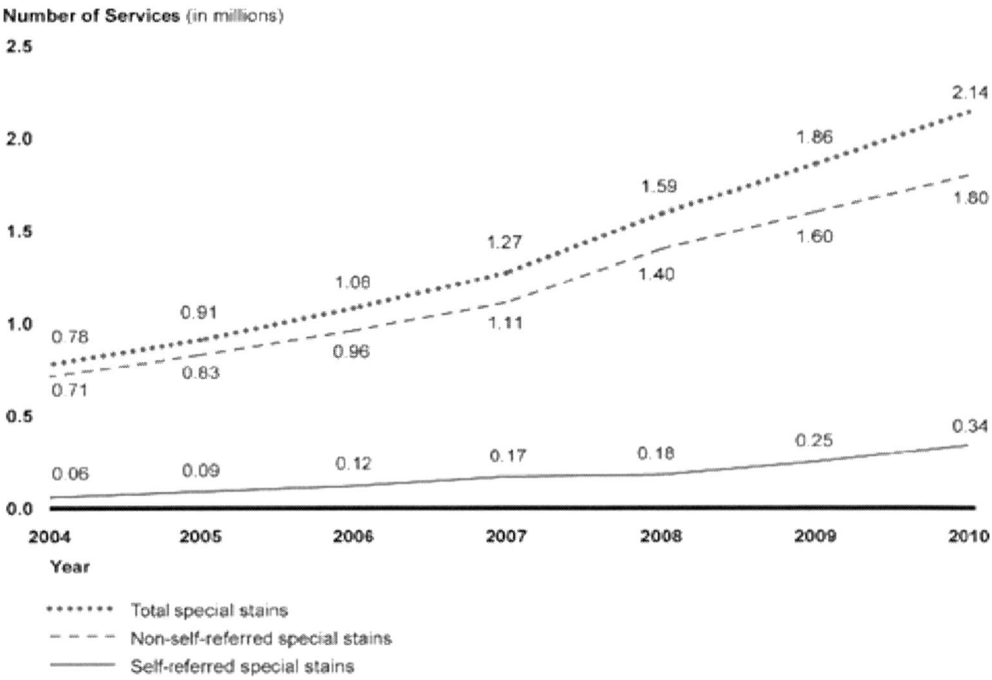

Source: GAO analysis of CMS data.

Note: Results include special stains—those services with Healthcare Common Procedure Coding System (HCPCS) codes of 88312, 88313, and 88342—that were performed in a physician's office or diagnostic laboratory and used in conjunction with the examination of tissue taken through biopsy procedures (HCPCS code 88305). Special stains performed in other settings, such as hospital outpatient departments, or performed with other anatomic pathology services are not included.

Figure 5. Number of Self-referred and Non-self-referred Medicare Special Stains, 2004–2010.

Similar to expenditures for anatomic pathology services, Medicare's expenditures for both self-referred and non-self-referred special stains used in conjunction with HCPCs code 88305 also grew rapidly during the period we studied, with the greater rate of increase among expenditures for self-referred services. Specifically, expenditures for self-referred special stains grew more than six-fold, increasing from about $4 million in 2004 to about $30 million in 2010 (see figure 6). In comparison, expenditures for non-self-referred special stains more than tripled during these years, growing from about $46 million in 2004 to about $162 million in 2010.

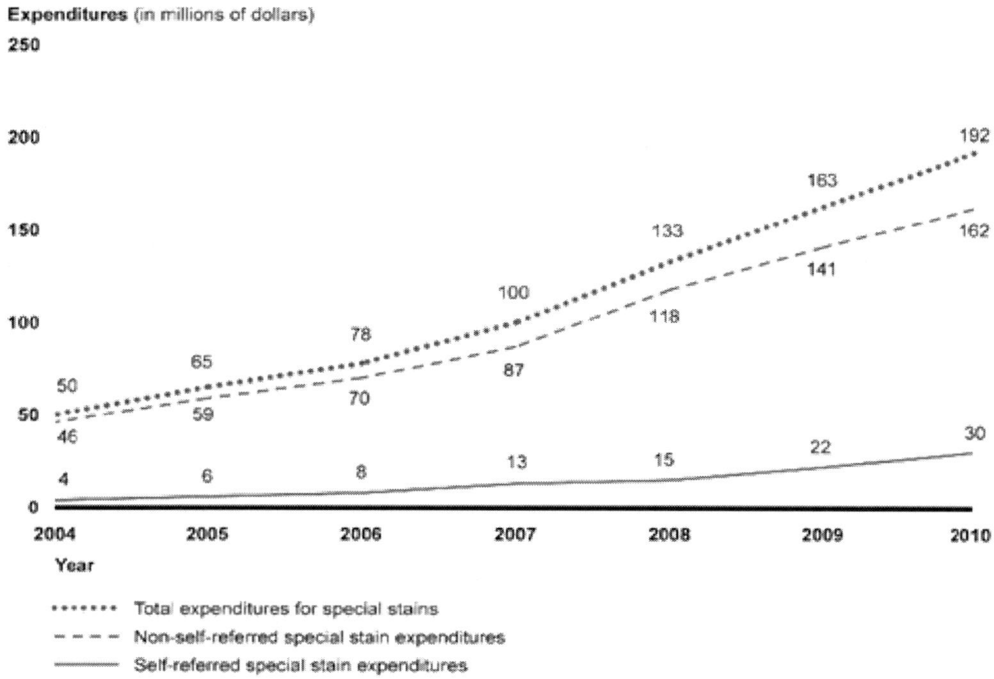

Source: GAO analysis of CMS data.

Note: Results include expenditures for special stains, those services with Healthcare Common Procedure Coding System (HCPCS) codes 88312, 88313, and 88342, performed in a physician's office or diagnostic laboratory that were performed with the anatomic pathology services (HCPCS code 88305) that are a focus of our study. Special stains performed in other settings, such as hospital outpatient departments, or performed with other anatomic pathology services are not included.

Figure 6. Expenditures for Self-referred and Non-self-referred Medicare Special Stains, 2004–2010.

Self-Referring and Non-Selfreferring Providers Referral for Special Stains

For two of the three specialties we examined, self-referring providers referred a higher number of special stains on average than non-selfreferring providers of the same specialty treating similar numbers of Medicare fee-for-service (FFS) beneficiaries. Specifically, self-referring gastroenterologists and urologists referred more special stains on average than non-self-referring gastroenterologists and urologists treating a similar number of Medicare beneficiaries. We also found this pattern for self-referring dermatologists treating small numbers of Medicare FFS beneficiaries. Provider specialty and size category combinations we studied where self-referring providers referred more special stains on average than non-self-referring providers represented about 86 percent of special stains referred by these specialties.

Table 6. Average Number of Medicare Special Stains Referred by Self-referring and Non-self-referring Providers for Select Provider Specialties in 2010

	Average number of special stains referred		
Provider specialty and number of unique Medicare FFS beneficiaries[a]	**Self-referring providers**	**Non-self-referring providers**	**Relative rate of self-referring providers[b]**
Dermatology			
1 to 250	17.6	15.3	1.15
251 to 500	32.8	36.8	0.89
>500	63.3	67.7	0.94
Gastroenterology			
1 to 250	73.4	44.2	1.66
251 to 500	201.9	119.4	1.69
>500	514.0	242.9	2.12
Urology			
1 to 250	17.0	12.6	1.35
251 to 500	36.3	31.8	1.14
>500	79.9	52.9	1.51

Source: GAO Analysis of CMS data.

Notes: Results include special stain HCPCS codes 88312, 88313, or 88342 used in conjunction with the anatomic pathology services we studied.

[a]The number of unique Medicare FFS beneficiaries refers to the number of unique beneficiaries that received at least one service from a provider.

[b]The relative rate of self-referring providers refers to the factor by which the average number of special stains referred by self-referring providers is greater or less than the average number of special stains referred by non-self-referring providers. For example, if the relative rate of self-referring providers is equal to 2, it would mean that, on average, self-referring providers referred twice as many special stains as non-self-referring providers.

Table 7. Change in Average Number of Medicare Special Stains Referred by Provider Specialty, 2008 and 2010

				Special stains[a]		
Primary specialty	Referral type	Number of providers	Average number of unique Medicare fee-for-service (FFS) beneficiaries, 2010	2008	2010	Percentage change 2008 to 2010
Dermatology	Switchers	130	478.2	31.2	36.7	17.6%
	Self-referring	1,353	573.6	31.1	35.9	15.4
	Non-self-referring	2,361	424.4	31.9	37.6	17.9
Gastroenterology	Switchers	195	335.5	125.9	219.3	74.2
	Self-referring	438	380.9	204.6	271.4	32.6
	Non-self-referring	4,833	365.1	99.3	119.0	19.8
Urology	Switchers	215	619.1	36.7	56.5	54.0
	Self-referring	498	626.8	27.5	38.8	41.1
	Non-self-referring	3,192	473.6	28.8	31.7	10.1

Source: GAO analysis of CMS data.

Notes: Special stains refer specifically to services with HCPCS codes 88312, 88313, or 88342. We define switchers as those providers that did not self-refer in 2007 or 2008, but did self-refer in 2009 and 2010.

[a]The average number of special stains referred by self-referring providers, non-self-referring providers, and switchers are influenced in part by the average number of unique Medicare FFS beneficiaries seen by each referral type. For example, in 2008, both switchers—who did not self-refer in 2008—and non-self-referring urologists averaged approximately 0.06 anatomic pathology referrals per unique Medicare FFS beneficiary. However, switchers averaged more anatomic pathology referrals than non-self-referring providers in 2008 because they saw, on average, more unique Medicare FFS beneficiaries.

Our analysis shows that, for two of the three specialties we reviewed, providers' referrals for special stains substantially increased the year after they began to self-refer. Specifically, urologists and gastroenterologists that were "switchers"—those providers that did not self-refer in 2007 or 2008 but began to self-refer in 2009 and continued to do so in 2010—saw larger increases in the number of special stain referrals they made relative to other providers (see table 7). Dermatologists in the switcher group had a 17.6 percent increase in the number of special stains referred from 2008 to 2010, but this was roughly equivalent to the increase for providers in the non-self-referring group and only slightly higher than the increase for providers in the self-referring group.

APPENDIX II: SCOPE AND METHODS

This section describes the scope and methodology used to analyze our three objectives: (1) trends in the number of and expenditures for self-referred and non-self-referred anatomic pathology services from 2004 through 2010, (2) how the provision of anatomic pathology services may differ for providers who self-refer when compared with other providers, and (3) the implications of self-referral for Medicare spending on anatomic pathology services.

For all three objectives, we used the Medicare Part B Carrier File, which contains final action Medicare Part B claims for noninstitutional providers, such as physicians. Claims can be for one or more services or for individual service components.[1] Each service or service component is identified on a claim by its Healthcare Common Procedure Coding System (HCPCS) code, which the Centers for Medicare & Medicaid Services (CMS) assigns to products, supplies, and services for billing purposes.

We limited our universe of services and service components for our study to certain anatomic pathology services. Specifically, we limited our universe to services with a HCPCS code of 88305, which are anatomic pathology services related to the examination of tissue taken through biopsy procedures. (We also studied services with HCPCS codes 88312, 88313, and 88342—special stains—which were used in conjunction with these anatomic pathology services.)[2] CMS considers anatomic pathology services to be "designated health services"—services for which, in the absence of an exception, a physician may not make a referral to an entity with which he or she has a financial relationship without implicating the Stark law.[3]

Because there is no indicator or "flag" on the claim that identifies whether services were self-referred or non-self-referred, we developed a claims-based methodology to identify services as either self-referred or non-selfreferred. Specifically, we classified services as self-referred if the provider that referred the beneficiary for an anatomic pathology service and the provider that performed the anatomic pathology service was identical or had a financial relationship. We used taxpayer identification number (TIN), an identification number used by the Internal Revenue Service, to determine providers' financial relationships. The TIN could be that of the provider, the provider's employer, or another entity to which the provider reassigns payment.[4] In order to identify the associated TINs for the referring and performing providers, we created a crosswalk of the performing provider's unique physician identification number or national provider identifier (NPI) to the TIN that appeared on the claim and used that to assign TINs to the referring and performing providers.[5]

We considered global services and separately-billed TCs to be self-referred if one or more of the TINs of the referring and performing provider matched. However, we did not consider separately-billed PCs to be self-referred, even if they met the same criterion. We did not count claims with PC only as self-referred because we could not reliably determine whether they corresponded to anatomic pathology services that were performed in a provider's office or laboratory. Further, we excluded claims where a HCPCS code of 88305 was billed with another anatomic pathology service and a special stain, because we could not determine which service required the use of the special stain. As part of developing this claims-based methodology to identify self-referred services, we interviewed officials from CMS, provider groups, and other researchers.

To describe the trends in the number of and expenditures for self-referred anatomic pathology services from 2004 through 2010, we used the Medicare Part B Carrier file to calculate utilization and expenditures for self-referred and non-self-referred anatomic pathology services, both in aggregate and per beneficiary. We limited this portion of our analysis to global claims or claims for a separately-billed TC for anatomic pathology services, which indicates that the performance of the anatomic pathology service was billed under the physician fee schedule. As a result, the universe for this portion of our analysis is those anatomic pathology services performed in a provider's office or in an independent clinical laboratory that both bill for the performance of an anatomic pathology service under the physician fee schedule. We focused on these settings because the financial incentive for providers to self-refer is most direct when the service is performed in a physician office. Further, we limited our analysis to self-referral of the preparation—as opposed to the interpretation—of these services, because we could determine the site of service as a physician's office or laboratory. Accordingly, we did not examine self-referral of the interpretation of these services as we could not reliably determine their site of service. Approximately two-thirds of all anatomic pathology services billed under the physician fee schedule were performed in a physician's office or clinical laboratory. To calculate the number of Medicare beneficiaries from 2004 through 2010 needed for per beneficiary calculations, we used the Denominator File, a database that contains enrollment information for all Medicare beneficiaries enrolled in a given year. We also examined the utilization for self-referred anatomic pathology services by provider specialty for 2004 and 2010.

To determine the extent to which the provision of anatomic pathology services differs for providers who self-refer when compared with other providers, we first classified providers based on the type of referrals they made. Specifically, we classified providers as self-referring if they self-referred at least one beneficiary for an anatomic pathology service.[6] We classified providers as non-self-referring if they referred a beneficiary for an anatomic pathology service, but did not self-refer any of the services. We assigned to each provider the anatomic pathology services, including those for the performance of an anatomic pathology service and those for the interpretation of the anatomic pathology service result. If the TC and PC were billed separately for the same beneficiary, we counted these two components as one referred service. As a result, we counted all services that a provider referred, regardless of whether it was performed in a provider office, independent clinical laboratory, or other setting. We classified anatomic pathology services as being from the same biopsy procedure if the services were referred by the same provider for the same beneficiary on the same day.[7] We then performed two separate analyses.

First, we compared the provision—that is, the number of referrals made— of anatomic pathology services by self-referring providers and non-selfreferring providers in 2010, disaggregated by the number of Medicare beneficiaries seen by the provider, provider specialty, and geography (i.e., urban or rural) and patient characteristics. We used the number of unique Medicare fee-for-service (FFS) beneficiaries for which providers provided services in 2010 as a proxy for practice size, which we identified using 100 percent of providers' claims from the Medicare Part B Carrier file. We defined urban settings as metropolitan statistical areas, a geographic entity defined by the Office of Management and Budget as a core urban area of 50,000 or more population. We used rural-urban commuting area codes—a Census tract-based classification scheme that utilizes the standard Bureau of Census Urbanized Area and Urban Cluster definitions in combination with work commuting information to characterize all of the nation's Census tracts regarding their rural and urban status—to identify providers as practicing in metropolitan statistical areas.[8] We considered all other settings to be rural. We identified providers' specialties on the basis of the specialties listed on the claims. These specialty codes include physician specialties, such as dermatology and urology, and nonphysician provider types, such as nurse practitioners and physician assistants. We also examined the extent to which the characteristics of the patient populations served by self-referring and nonself-referring providers differed. We used CMS's risk score file to identify average risk score, which serves as a proxy for beneficiary health status. Information on additional patient characteristics, such as age and sex, came from the Medicare Part B Carrier file claims.

Second, we determined the extent to which the number of anatomic pathology service referrals made by providers changed after they began to self-refer. Specifically, we identified a group of providers that began to self-refer anatomic pathology services in 2009. 9 We refer to this group of providers as "switchers" because it represents providers that did not self-refer in 2007 or 2008, but did self-refer in 2009 and 2010. We then calculated the change in the number of anatomic pathology referrals made from 2008 (i.e., the year before the switchers began self-referring) to 2010 (i.e., the year after they began self-referring). We compared the change in the number of referrals made by these providers to the change in the number of referrals made over the same time period by providers who did not change whether or not they self-referred anatomic pathology services. Specifically, we compared the change in the number of referrals made by switchers to those made by (1) self-referring providers—providers that self-referred in years 2007 through 2010, and (2) non-selfreferring providers—providers that did not self-refer in years 2007 through 2010. For each provider, we also identified the most common TIN to which they referred anatomic pathology services. If the TIN was the same for all 4 years, we assumed that they remained part of the same practice for all 4 years. We calculated the number of referrals in 2008 and 2010 separately for providers that met this criterion.

To determine the implications of self-referral for Medicare spending on anatomic pathology services, we summed the number of and expenditures for all anatomic pathology services performed in 2010 across the three provider specialties we reviewed. We then calculated the number of and expenditures for anatomic pathology services if self-referring providers performed biopsy procedures at the same rate as and referred the same number of services per biopsy procedure as non-selfreferring providers of the same provider size and specialty. We repeated this analysis incorporating an approximation of the payment reduction for anatomic pathology services that became effective in 2013.

We took several steps to ensure that the data used to produce this report were sufficiently reliable. Specifically, we assessed the reliability of the CMS data we used by interviewing officials responsible for overseeing these data sources, including CMS and Medicare contractor officials. We also reviewed relevant documentation, and examined the data for obvious errors, such as missing values and values outside of expected ranges. We determined that the data were sufficiently reliable for the purposes of our study, as they are used by the Medicare program as a record of payments to health care providers. As such, they are subject to routine CMS scrutiny.

We conducted this performance audit from January 2012 through June 2013 in accordance with generally accepted government auditing standards. Those standards require that we plan and perform the audit to obtain sufficient, appropriate evidence to provide a reasonable basis for our findings and conclusions based on our audit objectives. We believe that the evidence obtained provides a reasonable basis for our findings and conclusions based on our audit objectives.

Appendix III: Average Number of Medicare Anatomic Pathology Services per Biopsy Procedure for Most Common Diagnoses

Table 8. Average Number of Medicare Anatomic Pathology Services per Biopsy Procedure for Most Common Diagnoses Referred by Self-referring and Non-self-referring Dermatologists in 2010

Provider specialty and most common diagnoses, including International Classification of Diseases, Ninth Revision, Clinical Modification (ICD-9-CM) diagnostic code	Average number of anatomic pathology services per biopsy procedure		Percentage difference
	Self-referring providers	Non-self-referring providers	
Neoplasm of uncertain behavior of skin (238.2)	1.8	1.6	13%
Other malignant neoplasm of skin of other and unspecified parts of face (173.3)	1.6	1.4	14
Actinic keratosis (702.0)	1.7	1.5	13
Inflamed seborrheic keratosis (702.11)	1.6	1.4	14

Provider specialty and most common diagnoses, including International Classification of Diseases, Ninth Revision, Clinical Modification (ICD-9-CM) diagnostic code	Average number of anatomic pathology services per biopsy procedure		Percentage difference
	Self-referring providers	Non-self-referring providers	
Other malignant neoplasm of skin of upper limb, including shoulder (173.6)	1.6	1.4	14
Other seborrheic keratosis (702.19)	1.6	1.4	14
Other malignant neoplasm of skin of trunk, except scrotum (173.5)	1.6	1.5	7
Other malignant neoplasm of scalp and skin of neck (173.4)	1.6	1.5	7
Benign neoplasm of skin of trunk, except scrotum (216.5)	1.6	1.4	14
Neoplasm of unspecified nature of bone, soft tissue, and skin (239.2)	1.8	1.7	6
Scar conditions and fibrosis of skin (709.2)	1.6	1.4	14
Other malignant neoplasm of skin of lower limb, including hip (173.7)	1.6	1.4	14
Benign neoplasm of skin of other and unspecified parts of face (216.3)	1.6	1.4	14
Other malignant neoplasm of skin of ear and external auditory canal (173.2)	1.6	1.4	14
Contact dermatitis and other eczema unspecified cause (692.9)	1.4	1.2	17
Unspecified disorder of skin and subcutaneous tissue (709.9)	1.6	1.7	-6
Other malignant neoplasm of skin, site unspecified (173.9)	1.6	1.4	14
Benign neoplasm of skin, site unspecified (216.9)	1.6	1.4	14
Carcinoma in situ of skin of other and unspecified parts of face (232.3)	1.8	1.5	20
Viral warts, unspecified (078.10)	1.5	1.3	15
Other dyschromia (709.09)	1.6	1.4	14
Carcinoma in situ of skin of upper limb, including shoulder (232.6)	1.8	1.5	20

Source: GAO analysis of CMS data.

Note: All diagnoses that represent at least 1 percent of the principal diagnoses listed on the claims of self-referring dermatologists are included. Diagnoses are presented in order of the most to least common.

Table 9. Average Number of Medicare Anatomic Pathology Services per Biopsy Procedure for Most Common Diagnoses Referred by Self-referring and Non-self-referring Gastroenterologists in 2010

Provider specialty and most common diagnoses, including International Classification of Diseases, Ninth Revision, Clinical Modification (ICD-9-CM) diagnostic code	Average number of anatomic pathology services per biopsy procedure		Percentage difference
	Self-referring providers	Non-self-referring providers	
Benign neoplasm of colon (211.3)	2.2	1.9	16%
Atrophic gastritis, without mention of hemorrhage (535.10)	2.2	1.9	16

Table 9. (Continued)

Provider specialty and most common diagnoses, including International Classification of Diseases, Ninth Revision, Clinical Modification (ICD-9-CM) diagnostic code	Average number of anatomic pathology services per biopsy procedure		Percentage difference
	Self-referring providers	Non-self-referring providers	
Unspecified gastritis and gastroduodenitis, without mention of hemorrhage (535.50)	2.7	2.0	35
Other specified gastritis, without mention of hemorrhage (535.40)	2.3	1.9	21
Barrett's esophagus (530.85)	2.5	2.0	25
Benign neoplasm of stomach (211.1)	2.8	2.1	33
Benign neoplasm of rectum and anal canal (211.4)	1.9	1.6	19
Other and unspecified noninfectious gastroenteritis and colitis (558.9)	2.5	2.2	14
Diarrhea (787.91)	2.5	2.0	25
Unspecified disorder of stomach and duodenum (537.9)	2.3	2.1	10
Esophageal reflux (530.81)	2.6	2.0	30
Reflux esophagitis (530.11)	2.4	2.0	20
Esophagitis, unspecified (530.10)	2.0	1.8	11
Acute gastritis, without mention of hemorrhage (535.00)	2.3	2.0	15
Other specified disorders of stomach and duodenum (537.89)	2.3	1.9	21
Dysphagia, unspecified (787.20)	2.3	1.7	35
Anal and rectal polyp (569.0)	1.9	1.5	27
Other specified disorders of intestine (569.89)	2.3	1.8	28
Duodenitis, without mention of hemorrhage (535.60)	3.0	2.5	20

Source: GAO analysis of CMS data.

Note: All diagnoses that represent at least 1 percent of the principal diagnoses listed on the claims of self-referring gastroenterologists are included. Diagnoses are presented in order of the most to least common.

Table 10. Average Number of Medicare Anatomic Pathology Services per Biopsy Procedure for Most Common Diagnoses Referred by Self-referring and Non-self-referring Urologists in 2010

Provider specialty and most common diagnoses, including International Classification of Diseases, Ninth Revision, Clinical Modification (ICD-9-CM) diagnostic code	Average number of anatomic pathology services per biopsy procedure		Percentage difference
	Self-referring providers	Non-self-referring providers	
Elevated prostate specific antigen (790.93)	12.5	8.5	47%
Malignant neoplasm of prostate (185)	8.5	6.1	39
Malignant neoplasm of bladder, part unspecified (188.9)	1.8	1.7	6
Hyperplasia of prostate, unspecified, without urinary obstruction and other lower urinary symptoms (LUTS) (600.90)	5.0	3.2	56
Other chronic cystitis (595.2)	1.8	1.7	6

Provider specialty and most common diagnoses, including International Classification of Diseases, Ninth Revision, Clinical Modification (ICD-9-CM) diagnostic code	Average number of anatomic pathology services per biopsy procedure: Self-referring providers	Non-self-referring providers	Percentage difference
Hypertrophy (benign) of prostate without urinary obstruction and other lower urinary tract symptom (LUTS) (600.00)	5.3	2.6	104
Hypertrophy (benign) of prostate with urinary obstruction and other lower urinary tract symptoms (LUTS) (600.01)	3.1	2.3	35
Benign neoplasm of prostate (222.2)	9.4	6.6	42
Hematuria, unspecified (599.70)	1.9	1.4	36
Carcinoma in situ of prostate (233.4)	11.5	7.6	51
Nodular prostate without urinary obstruction (600.10)	7.6	5.0	52
Chronic prostatitis (601.1)	6.1	4.4	39
Cystitis, unspecified (595.9)	1.8	1.6	13

Source: GAO analysis of CMS data.

Note: All diagnoses that represent at least 1 percent of the principal diagnoses listed on the claims of self-referring urologists are included. Diagnoses are listed in order of the most to least common.

Appendix IV: Age and Sex of Medicare Beneficiaries for Select Provider Specialties by Practice Size in 2010

Table 11. Average Age of Medicare Beneficiaries for Select Provider Specialties by Practice Size in 2010

Provider specialty and number of unique Medicare FFS beneficiaries[a]	Average age (in years) of beneficiaries: Self-referring providers	Non-self-referring providers
Dermatology		
1 to 250	73	73
251 to 500	74	74
> 500	74	74
Gastroenterology		
1 to 250	67	70
251 to 500	70	71
> 500	71	71
Urology		
1 to 250	70	71
251 to 500	72	73
> 500	74	73

Source: GAO analysis of CMS data.

[a]The number of unique Medicare FFS beneficiaries refers to the number of unique beneficiaries that received at least one service from a provider.

Table 12. Average Percentage of Medicare Beneficiaries Who Are Female for Select Provider Specialties by Practice Size in 2010

	Average percentage of beneficiaries female	
Provider specialty and number of unique Medicare FFS beneficiaries[a]	**Self-referring providers**	**Non-self-referring providers**
Dermatology		
1 to 250	51	53
251 to 500	51	52
> 500	51	52
Gastroenterology		
1 to 250	58	57
251 to 500	57	57
> 500	57	58
Urology		
1 to 250	30	30
251 to 500	28	28
> 500	25	25

Source: GAO analysis of CMS data.

[a] The number of unique Medicare FFS beneficiaries refers to the number of unique beneficiaries that received at least one service from a provider.

APPENDIX V: AVERAGE NUMBER OF MEDICARE ANATOMIC PATHOLOGY REFERRALS BY PROVIDER SELF-REFERRAL AND URBAN-RURAL STATUS IN 2010

		Average number of anatomic pathology services		
Geographic designation	Provider specialty and number of unique Medicare fee-for-service (FFS) beneficiaries[a]	Self-referring providers	Non-self-referring providers	Relative rate of self-referring providers[b]
Urban	Dermatology			
	1 to 250	168.7	142.5	1.18
	251 to 500	538.0	445.1	1.21
	>500	1,532.1	1,019.4	1.50
	Gastroenterology			
	1 to 250	174.9	139.0	1.26
	251 to 500	414.9	344.2	1.21
	>500	800.5	628.6	1.27
	Urology			
	1 to 250	96.9	74.4	1.30
	251 to 500	250.4	171.9	1.46
	>500	472.8	299.3	1.58
Rural	Dermatology			
	1 to 250	183.0	166.2	1.10
	251 to 500	570.7	510.7	1.12
	>500	1,863.3	939.0	1.99
	Gastroenterology			

Geographic designation	Provider specialty and number of unique Medicare fee-for-service (FFS) beneficiaries[a]	Average number of anatomic pathology services		
		Self-referring providers	Non-self-referring providers	Relative rate of self-referring providers[b]
	1 to 250	114.3	185.9	0.61
	251 to 500	478.8	403.1	1.19
	>500	963.4	726.3	1.33
	Urology			
	1 to 250	142.5	83.5	1.71
	251 to 500	206.3	188.2	1.10
	>500	373.9	316.2	1.18

Source: GAO analysis of CMS data.

Notes: Anatomic pathology services refer specifically to Healthcare Common Procedure Coding System (HCPCS) code 88305. Providers were considered to be self-referring if they self-referred anatomic pathology services for at least one biopsy procedure. Of the 29,502 providers represented above that referred at least one beneficiary for an anatomic pathology service in 2010, 7,109 were self-referring and 22,393 were non-self-referring.

[a] The number of unique Medicare FFS beneficiaries refers to the number of unique beneficiaries that received at least one service from a provider.

[b] The relative rate of self-referring providers refers to the factor by which the average number of services referred by self-referring providers is greater or less than the average number of services referred by non-self-referring providers. For example, if the relative rate of self-referring providers is equal to 2, it would mean that, on average, self-referring providers referred twice as many anatomic pathology services as non-self-referring providers.

End Notes

[1] Compliance with the physician self-referral law, commonly known as the Stark law, is outside the scope of this report. The Stark law prohibits physicians from making referrals for certain designated health services paid for by Medicare, to entities with which the physicians or immediate family members have a financial relationship, unless the arrangement complies with a specified exception, such as in-office ancillary services. 42 U.S.C. § 1395nn(b)(2). The requirements of the in-office ancillary services exception are found at 42 C. F. R. § 411.355(b) (2012).

[2] Anatomic pathology includes multiple subspecialties, such as surgical pathology—the macroscopic and microscopic examination of surgical specimens; cytopathology—the examination of cells from fluids or smears; and hematology—the examination of cells from bone marrow aspirations or biopsies. For the purposes of this report "anatomic pathology" services refer to those services with a Healthcare Common Procedure Coding System (HCPCS) code of 88305.

[3] For studies by GAO and other agencies on physician self-referral, see, for example, GAO, *Medicare: Higher Use of Advanced Imaging Services by Providers Who Self-Refer Costing Medicare Millions*, GAO-12-966 (Washington, D.C.: Sept. 28, 2012) and Medicare Payment Advisory Commission, *Report to the Congress: Improving Incentives in the Medicare Program* (Washington, D.C.: June 2009). For studies by HHS OIG on physician self-referral of anatomic pathology services, see Department of Health and Human Services, Office of the Inspector General, *Audit of Pathology Laboratory Services Claimed by Florida Urology Physicians, P.A. for the Period September through December 2004* (Washington, D.C.: June 2007); *Review of Pathology Services Claimed by Urology Tyler, P.A. Tyler, Texas from May Through December 2004* (Washington, D.C.: June 2007); and *Audit of Pathology Laboratory Services Claimed by Atlantic Urological Associates, P.A. for Calendar Year 2004* (Washington, D.C., June 2007).

[4] In addition to this report on anatomic pathology services, we have ongoing work related to the self-referral of intensity-modulated radiation therapy services and physical therapy services.

[5] An indicator or "flag" could be, for example, a modifier that a provider lists on a claim to indicate that a service is self-referred. Providers currently use modifiers to provide additional information about a service to CMS. For example, if a provider is only billing for the technical component of an anatomic pathology service, the provider would use a modifier to alert CMS that the claim does not cover the professional component of the service.

[6] Providers could have a financial relationship with the same entity if, for example, they are part of the same group practice.

[7] We use the term "biopsy procedure" to refer to the process of extracting tissue samples for analysis. Multiple tissue samples (sometimes also referred to as biopsies) can be extracted from a single biopsy procedure.

[8] Providers can also provide anatomic pathology services in settings other than physician offices or clinical laboratories, such as hospitals.

[9] We did not analyze the self-referral related to the interpretation of these services because we could not reliably determine whether they were performed in a physician's office or independent laboratory using Medicare Part B Carrier File data.

[10] We defined urban settings as metropolitan statistical areas, a geographic entity defined by the Office of Management and Budget as a core urban area of 50,000 or more in population; all other settings are considered rural.

[11] We used 4 years of experience (2007 through 2010) to categorize providers even though we compared referrals in 2008 to 2010 because we wanted to ensure that providers that began self-referring in 2009 did not self-refer for at least the 2 prior years.

[12] See *Medicare Program; Revision of Payment Policies Under the Physician Fee Schedule for CY 2013*, 77 Fed. Reg. 68,892 (Nov. 16, 2012).

[13] Key types of skin biopsy procedures include (1) shave (use of a tool to remove a small section of the top layers of the skin), (2) punch (use of a circular tool to remove a small section of the skin), and (3) excisional (use of a scalpel to remove an entire area of abnormal skin).

[14] Specifically, billing providers under these arrangements are limited in the amount they can charge Medicare for the cost of leasing equipment and contracting with staff to perform the service when the services are purchased from other providers or performed at a site other than where the full range of physician services is provided. See *Medicare Program: Revisions to Payment Policies under the Physician Fee Schedule and Other Part B Payment Policies for CY 2008*. 72 Fed. Reg. 66,222. (Nov. 27, 2007) (amending 42 C.F.R. § 414.50).

[15] *Medicare Program; Payment Policies Under the Physician Fee Schedule for CY 2009*, 73 Fed. Reg. 69,726 (Nov. 19, 2008) (amending 42 C.F.R. § 414.50). Under this rule, a shared practice exists if either (1) the performing physician furnishes at least 75 percent of his or her services through the billing provider, or (2) the physician performs or conducts and supervises a diagnostic test in the office of the billing provider.

[16] 73 Fed. Reg. 69,726, 69,751 (Nov. 19, 2008). CMS made this change after concluding that anatomic pathology services resulting from prostate saturation biopsies did not require the same amount of provider work in terms of evaluation, interpretation, and reporting as other anatomic pathology services.

[17] In the 2013 physician fee schedule, CMS revised HCPCS G4016 to payment for 10 to 20 specimens. See *Medicare Program; Revisions to Payment Policies Under the Physician Fee Schedule,* 77 Fed. Reg. 68,892 (Nov. 16, 2012).

[18] For example, on the basis of 2009 payment rates, a provider that performed both the TC and PC for 30 anatomic pathology services resulting from a prostate saturation biopsy procedure was paid about $1,233 under G0417. However, if a provider was paid at the 2009 payment rate for HCPCS code 88305 for each of the 30 services, he or she would have received about $3,116.

[19] See *Medicare Program; Revision of Payment Policies under the Physician Fee Schedule for CY 2013*, 77 Fed. Reg. 68,892 (Nov. 16, 2012). This estimate of the 2013 payment reduction does not include payment reductions that may result from implementation of the Budget Control Act of 2011, Pub. L. No. 112-25, 125 Stat. 240, as amended by the American Taxpayer Relief Act of 2012 (Pub. L. No. 112-240, 126 Stat. 2313) (2013).

[20] Payment for these services include expenditures beneficiaries paid as part of cost-sharing paid under Medicare.

[21] While the total number of Medicare beneficiaries increased during our study period, the number of beneficiaries enrolled in Medicare FFS decreased. This was due to increased enrollment in the Medicare Advantage program, an alternative to the original Medicare FFS program in which private health plans offer health care coverage to Medicare beneficiaries.

[22] This increase in 2009 corresponds to CMS's identification of an exception to the anti-markup rule implemented in 2008. *See Medicare Program; Payment Policies Under the Physician Fee Schedule for CY 2009*, 73 Fed. Reg. 69,726 (Nov. 19, 2008) (amending 42 C.F.R. § 414.50).

[23] We classified anatomic pathology services as being from the same biopsy procedure if they were referred by the same provider, for the same beneficiary, on the same day.

[24] We examined the number of services referred per biopsy procedure for each diagnosis that comprised at least 1 percent of the diagnoses listed on the claims referred by self-referring providers for each of the three provider specialties. The one primary diagnosis for which self-referring providers did not refer more services per biopsy procedure on average than non-self-referring providers was unspecified disorder of skin and subcutaneous tissue (709.9). This diagnosis accounted for approximately 1.6 percent of the diagnoses listed on claims for self-referring dermatologists.

[25] A risk score is a relative measure of a beneficiary's expected health care costs and serves as a proxy for a beneficiary's health status.

[26] We limited our analysis to expenditures directly related to anatomic pathology services. There may be additional costs associated with the increased use of anatomic pathology services by self-referring providers, if these services result in inaccurate diagnoses and, in turn, additional services or procedures that are unnecessary. In contrast, increased use of anatomic pathology services may partially offset some of these direct anatomic pathology costs if increased use led to the early detection of disease and resulted in less-invasive and less-costly treatments.

[27] See Medicare Payment Advisory Commission: Report to the Congress: Improving Incentives in the Medicare Program (Washington, DC, June 2009).

End Note for Appendix I

[1] This special stain (88342 – immunohistochemistry) is used to evaluate diseases, including diagnosis, staging, and prognosis. For example, immunohistochemistry can be used to detect whether the specimen where cancer has been found is the primary site of that cancer or whether the cancer has spread to that location from elsewhere in the body.

End Notes for Appendix II

[1] Services can have technical components (TC) and professional components (PC). The TC of a service is intended to cover the performance of a test, including the cost of equipment, supplies, and nonphysician staff. The PC of the service is intended to cover the physician's time in interpreting an anatomic pathology service and writing a report on the findings. The TC and PC of a service can be billed together on the same claim—called a global claim—or billed separately.

[2] For the purposes of this report "anatomic pathology" services refer to HCPCS 88305 services, and "special stains" refer to HCPCS 88312, 88313, and 88342 services that were used in conjunction with these anatomic pathology services.

[3] Compliance with the physician self-referral law, commonly known as the Stark law, is outside the scope of this report. The Stark law prohibits physicians from making referrals for certain designated health services paid for by Medicare to entities with which the physicians or immediate family members have a financial relationship, unless the arrangement complies with a specified exception, such as in-office ancillary services. 42 U.S.C. § 1395nn(b)(2).

[4] Some providers may be associated with TINs with which they do not have a direct or indirect financial relationship and thus would not have the same incentives as other self-referring providers. We anticipate that relatively few providers in our self-referring group meet this description but to the extent that they do, it may have limited the differences we found in utilization and expenditure rates between self-referring and non-self-referring providers.

[5] The final rule implementing the Health Insurance Portability and Accountability Act established the standard for a unique health identifier for health care providers for use in the health care system and announced the adoption of the NPI as that standard. *HIPAA Administrative Simplification: Standard Unique Health Identifier for*

Health Care Providers, 69 Fed. Reg. 2424 (Jan. 23, 2004) (adding a new subpart D to 45 C.F.R. part 162). Performing physicians were required to include their NPI on any claim submitted to Medicare as of May 23, 2008. Prior to implementation of the NPI, Medicare required providers to submit another type of unique provider identifier called the unique physician identification number. Our methodology for identifying self-referred services was similar to the methodology we used for our study of physician self-referral of imaging services. See GAO, *Medicare: Higher Use of Advanced Imaging Services by Providers Who Self-Refer Costing Medicare Millions*, GAO-12-966 (Washington, D.C.: Sept. 28, 2012).

[6] Providers in our analysis that could self-refer include primarily physicians, but also could include other providers, such as nurse practitioners and physician assistants.

[7] We use the term "biopsy procedure" to refer to the process of extracting tissue for analysis. Multiple tissue samples (sometimes also referred to as biopsies) can be extracted from a single biopsy procedure.

[8] We considered a location with a rural-urban commuting area code of 1.0, 1.1, 2.0, 2.1, or 3.0 to be a metropolitan statistical area.

[9] We used 4 years of experience (2007 through 2010) to categorize providers even though we compared referrals in 2008 to 2010 because we wanted to ensure that providers that began self-referring in 2009 did not self-refer for at least the 2 prior years.

In: Physician Self-Referrals
Editor: Louise Hamilton

ISBN: 978-1-63463-444-1

Chapter 4

MEDICARE: HIGHER USE OF ADVANCED IMAGING SERVICES BY PROVIDERS WHO SELF-REFER COSTING MEDICARE MILLIONS*

United States Government Accountability Office

ABBREVIATIONS

BETOS	Berenson-Eggers Type of Service
CMS	Centers for Medicare & Medicaid Services
CT	computed tomography
DRA	Deficit Reduction Act of 2005
FFS	fee-for-service
HCPCS	Healthcare Common Procedure Coding System
HHS	Department of Health and Human Services
IDTF	independent diagnostic testing facility
MedPAC	Medicare Payment Advisory Commission
MRI	magnetic resonance imaging
NPI	national provider identifier
PC	professional component
PPACA	Patient Protection and Affordable Care Act
TC	technical component
TIN	taxpayer identification number

* This is an edited, reformatted and augmented version of The United States Government Accountability Office publication, Report to Congressional Requesters, GAO-12-966, dated September 2012.

WHY GAO DID THIS STUDY

Medicare Part B expenditures—which include payment for advanced imaging services—are expected to continue growing at an unsustainable rate. Questions have been raised about selfreferral's role in this growth. Self-referral occurs when a provider refers patients to entities in which the provider or the provider's family members have a financial interest. GAO was asked to examine the prevalence of advanced imaging self-referral and its effect on Medicare spending. This report examines (1) trends in the number of and expenditures for self-referred and nonself-referred advanced imaging services, (2) how provision of these services differs among providers on the basis of whether they self-refer, and (3) implications of self-referral for Medicare spending. GAO analyzed Medicare Part B claims data from 2004 through 2010 and interviewed officials from the Centers for Medicare & Medicaid Services (CMS) and other stakeholders. Because Medicare claims lack an indicator identifying self-referred services, GAO developed a claims-based methodology to identify self-referred services and expenditures and to characterize providers as self-referring or not.

WHAT GAO RECOMMENDS

GAO recommends that CMS improve its ability to identify self-referral of advanced imaging services and address increases in these services. The Department of Health and Human Services, which oversees CMS, stated it would consider one recommendation, but did not concur with the others. GAO maintains CMS should monitor these self-referred services and ensure they are appropriate.

WHAT GAO FOUND

From 2004 through 2010, the number of self-referred and non-self-referred advanced imaging services—magnetic resonance imaging (MRI) and computed tomography (CT) services—both increased, with the larger increase among self-referred services. For example, the number of self-referred MRI services increased over this period by more than 80 percent, compared with an increase of 12 percent for non-self-referred MRI services. Likewise, the growth rate of expenditures for self-referred MRI and CT services was also higher than for nonself-referred MRI and CT services.

GAO's analysis showed that providers' referrals of MRI and CT services substantially increased the year after they began to self-refer—that is, they purchased or leased imaging equipment, or joined a group practice that already self-referred. Providers that began self-referring in 2009—referred to as switchers—increased MRI and CT referrals on average by about 67 percent in 2010 compared to 2008. In the case of MRIs, the average number of referrals switchers made increased from 25.1 in 2008 to 42.0 in 2010. In contrast, the average number of referrals made by providers who remained self-referrers or non-self-referrers declined during this period. This comparison suggests that the increase in the average number of referrals for switchers was not due to a general increase in the use of imaging services among all providers. GAO's examination of all providers that referred an MRI or CT service in 2010 showed that self-referring providers referred about two times as many of these services as providers who did not self-refer. Differences persisted after accounting for practice size, specialty, geography, or patient characteristics. These two analyses suggest that financial incentives for self-referring providers were likely a major factor driving the increase in referrals.

Change in Average Number of MRI Services Referred, 2008 and 2010

	Average 2008 referred MRI services	Average 2010 referred MRI services	Percentage change
Switchers	25.1	42.0	67.3
Non-self-referrers	20.6	19.2	-6.8
Self-referrers	47.0	45.4	-3.4

Source: GAO analysis of Medicare data.

Note: Pattern observed for MRI services was similar for CT services. GAO defines switchers as those providers that did not self-refer in 2007 or 2008, but did self-refer in 2009 and 2010.

GAO estimates that in 2010, providers who self-referred likely made 400,000 more referrals for advanced imaging services than they would have if they were not self-referring. These additional referrals cost Medicare about $109 million. To the extent that these additional referrals were unnecessary, they pose unacceptable risks for beneficiaries, particularly in the case of CT services, which involve the use of ionizing radiation that has been linked to an increased risk of developing cancer.

* * *

September 28, 2012

Congressional Requesters

Expenditures for Medicare Part B services—which include physician and other outpatient services—are expected to continue exceeding the overall growth rate of the U.S. economy, heightening concerns about the long-range fiscal sustainability of Medicare.[1] While Medicare spending growth has slowed in recent years, expenditures for Medicare Part B grew by an average of 5.9 percent annually from 2007 through 2011 and are projected to grow by an average of 7.6 percent annually from 2012 through 2016.[2] In comparison, the national economy grew by an average annual rate of 2.5 percent from 2007 through 2011[3] and is projected to increase on average by 4.6 percent annually from 2012 through 2016.[4] Medicare Part B spending includes payments for advanced imaging services—magnetic resonance imaging (MRI) and computed tomography (CT) services—which providers use in the diagnosis and treatment of many diseases and disorders, such as different types of cancer, cardiovascular diseases, and musculoskeletal disorders.[5]

Policymakers and researchers have raised questions about the growth in Part B spending, noting that some of this growth may be partially attributed to self-referral and that not all of the advanced imaging services provided may be appropriate or necessary.[6] Self-referral occurs when providers refer their patients to entities—such as themselves or a group practice—with which they or an immediate family member has a financial relationship, such as when a provider refers patients to his or her office for advanced imaging services after the provider purchases or leases advanced imaging equipment.[7] Proponents of self-referral point out that such arrangements allow providers to make rapid diagnoses, improve coordination of care, and provide convenient access for patients. However, critics of self-referral note that the incentive for financial gain in such arrangements may result in inappropriate, unnecessary, or potentially harmful services.

For example, CT services expose beneficiaries to ionizing radiation, which is associated with an increased risk of cancer.

Growth in imaging services expenditures—including expenditures for advanced imaging services—have prompted action from Congress and resulted in recommendations from us and others. Specifically, Congress, as part of the Deficit Reduction Act of 2005 (DRA), [8] required that Medicare payment for certain imaging services under the Medicare physician fee schedule—the payment system used to determine fees for physician-billed services in Medicare FFS—not exceed the amount Medicare pays under the hospital outpatient prospective payment system, used to pay for hospital outpatient services. In our 2008 report, we recommended that, to address the rapid growth in Medicare Part B imaging expenditures, the Centers for Medicare & Medicaid Services (CMS)—the agency within the Department of Health and Human Services that administers the Medicare program—examine the feasibility of expanding the use of front-end approaches for managing the utilization of advanced imaging services.[9]

Front-end approaches to managing services are conducted prior to, rather than after, services are performed and payment is made. Examples of such approaches include requiring prior authorization (specific approval from a payer to perform a service) and privileging (limiting the authority to order certain services to only providers with specified qualifications). In contrast, back-end approaches are used after CMS issues payment, and could include targeted audits of providers that refer a high volume of services. Further, the Medicare Payment Advisory Commission (MedPAC) has recommended that certain providers with higher advanced imaging utilization participate in a prior authorization program and that CMS reduce payment rates for imaging services when the same provider orders and performs a service.[10] According to MedPAC, such a reduction would account for certain efficiencies that occur when the same provider orders and performs a service. Specifically, in these situations, the provider has likely already performed certain work involved in interpreting an imaging service, such as reviewing the patient's history, prior to making the referral. As of June 2012, CMS has not implemented MedPAC's or our recommendation.

You asked us to examine the prevalence of self-referral for advanced imaging services and Medicare spending for these services.[11] In this report, we examine (1) trends in the number of and expenditures for self-referred and non-self-referred advanced imaging services from 2004 through 2010, (2) the extent to which the provision of advanced imaging services differs for providers who self-refer when compared with other providers, and (3) the implications of self-referral for Medicare spending on advanced imaging services.

To identify trends in the number of and expenditures for self-referred and non-self-referred advanced imaging services from 2004 through 2010, we analyzed claims from the Medicare Part B Carrier File for MRI and CT services.[12] Because there is no indicator or "flag" on the claim that identifies whether services are self-referred or non-self-referred and

CMS has no other method for identifying whether a service was self-referred, we developed a claims-based methodology for identifying self-referred services.[13]

Specifically, we classified services from the period we reviewed as self-referred if the provider that referred the beneficiary for a MRI or CT service and the provider that performed the MRI or CT service were identical or had a financial relationship with the same entity.[14] We removed MRI or CT services referred by radiologists or other providers that primarily practice in an independent diagnostic testing facility (IDTF) because they have limited ability to self-refer services.[15] We limited the universe for this portion of our analysis to those advanced imaging services performed in a provider's office or in an IDTF, which represents approximately one-fifth of all advanced imaging services provided to Medicare FFS beneficiaries.[16] Providers in our analysis include primarily physicians, but could include other providers, such as nurse practitioners and physician assistants. We focused on services performed in these settings because our previous work showed rapid growth among such services and because the financial incentive for providers to self-refer is most direct when the service is performed in a physician office. We used the claims to identify trends in the number and proportion of self-referred and non-self-referred MRI and CT services performed from 2004 through 2010, the expenditures for these services from 2004 through 2010, and the proportion of self-referred and non-self-referred MRI and CT services by provider specialty for 2004 and 2010. To determine expenditures, we used the allowed charges variable from the Medicare Part B Carrier File, which includes the amounts paid by Medicare and the beneficiary.

To determine the extent to which the provision of advanced imaging services differed for providers who self-refer when compared with other providers, we performed two separate analyses. First, we compared the provision—that is, the number of referrals made—of MRI and CT services by self-referring providers and non-self-referring providers in 2010, after accounting for factors such as practice size (i.e., the number of Medicare beneficiaries), provider specialty, geography (i.e., urban or rural), and patient characteristics. [17] For this analysis, our universe of providers included all those providers that referred at least one MRI or CT service, except for providers that had a specialty of radiology, emergency medicine, or provided services in an IDTF.[18] Second, we determined the extent to which the number of MRI and CT referrals made by providers changed after they began to self-refer. Specifically, we identified a groupof providers that began to self-refer advanced imaging services in 2009. We then calculated the change in the number of MRI or CT referrals made from 2008 (i.e., the year before they began self-referring) to 2010 (i.e., the year after they began self-referring).

We compared the change in the number of referrals made by these providers to the change in the number of referrals made over the same time period by providers who did not change whether or not they self-referred advanced imaging services. We classified providers as self-referring if they self-referred at least one MRI or CT service and non-self-referring if they referred—but did not selfrefer—at least one MRI or CT service.[19] For both analyses we counted all services that a provider referred, regardless of whether it was performed in a provider office, IDTF, or other setting, such as a hospital.

To determine the implications of self-referral for Medicare spending on advanced imaging services, we estimated what Medicare expenditures under the physician fee schedule for self-referred advanced imaging services would have been in 2010 if the rate of referrals made by self-referring providers equaled the rate of referrals made by providers who did not self-refer.

We compared this to the actual expenditures under the physician fee schedule, using the allowed charges variable, for self-referred advanced imaging services of the same specialty and provider size and calculated the difference. To ensure comparisons were meaningful, we limited this analysis to providers in those specialties that had at least 1,000 self-referring providers. [20]

We took several steps to ensure that the data used to produce this report were sufficiently reliable.

Specifically, we assessed the reliability of the CMS data we used by interviewing officials responsible for overseeing these data sources, reviewing relevant documentation, and examining the data for obvious errors. We determined that the data were sufficiently reliable for the purposes of our study. (See app. I for more details on our scope and methodology.)

We conducted this performance audit from May 2010 through September 2012 in accordance with generally accepted government auditing standards. Those standards require that we plan and perform the audit to obtain sufficient, appropriate evidence to provide a reasonable basis for our findings and conclusions based on our audit objectives. We believe that the evidence obtained provides a reasonable basis for our findings and conclusions based on our audit objectives.

BACKGROUND

MRI and CT services are two types of medical imaging that aid in the diagnosis and treatment of myriad diseases and disorders. Medicare reimburses providers for performing the services and, subsequently, interpreting the results. Payment for the performance of the service can be made through different payment systems, depending on where the service is performed.

In 2010, 6.8 million MRI and CT services were performed in a physician office or IDTF, representing about 23 percent of all MRI and CT services received by Medicare FFS beneficiaries. CMS has implemented several policies to limit self-referral, and MedPAC and other researchers have proposed further reforms.

MRI and CT Services

Medical imaging is a noninvasive process used to obtain pictures of the internal anatomy or function of the anatomy using one of many different types of imaging equipment and media for creating the image. MRI and CT services are two of the six medical imaging modalities.[21] MRI services use magnets, radio waves, and computers to create images of internal body tissues. CT services use ionizing radiation and computers to produce cross-sectional images of internal organs and body structures. For certain advanced imaging services, contrast agents, such as barium or iodine solutions, are administered to patients orally or intravenously.

By using contrast, sometimes referred to as "dye," as part of the imaging examination, providers can view soft tissue and organ function more clearly. MRI and CT services help diagnose and treat many diseases and disorders such as different types of cancer, cardiovascular diseases, and musculoskeletal disorders.

They can also reduce the need for more-invasive medical procedures and improve patient outcomes.

Medicare Billing and Payment Policies for Advanced Imaging Services

Medicare payments for advanced imaging services are separated into two components—the technical component (TC) and the professional component (PC). The TC is intended to cover the cost of performing a test, including the costs for equipment, supplies, and nonphysician staff. The PC is intended to cover the provider's time in interpreting the image and writing a report on the findings. The PC and TC can be billed together, on what is called a global claim.

The components can also be billed separately. For instance, a global claim could be billed if the same provider performs and interprets the examination, whereas the TC and PC could be billed separately if the performing and interpreting providers are different. Typically, the Medicare payment for the TC is substantially higher than the payment for the PC. For instance, for a CT of the pelvis with dye billed under the 2010 Medicare physician fee schedule, the TC accounted for 79 percent of the total payment, and the PC accounted for 21 percent.

Medicare reimburses providers through different payment systems depending on where the advanced imaging service is performed. When an advanced imaging service is performed in a provider's office or an IDTF, both the PC and TC are reimbursed under the Medicare physician fee schedule.

Alternatively, when the service is performed in an institutional setting, such as a hospital outpatient or inpatient department, the provider is reimbursed under the Medicare physician fee schedule for the PC, while the TC is reimbursed under a different Medicare payment system, according to the setting in which the service was provided. For instance, the TC of an advanced imaging service performed in a hospital outpatient department is reimbursed under the Medicare hospital outpatient payment system, while a service performed in a hospital inpatient setting is reimbursed through a facility payment paid under Medicare Part A.

2010 Advanced Imaging Utilization by Setting and Medicare Physician Fee Schedule Expenditures

In 2010, Medicare FFS beneficiaries received 30.0 million advanced imaging services, approximately 6.8 million (23 percent) of which were performed in an IDTF or physician's office.

Of the 6.8 million advanced imaging services performed in an IDTF or physician's office, 2.9 million were MRI services and 3.9 million were CT services. The remaining 23.2 million advanced imaging services were performed in other settings, such as hospital inpatient or outpatient departments, and their associated TCs were billed through different payment systems (see figure 1).

The total expenditures for all advanced imaging services billed under the Medicare physician fee schedule, including TCs and PCs, reached $4.2 billion in 2010.

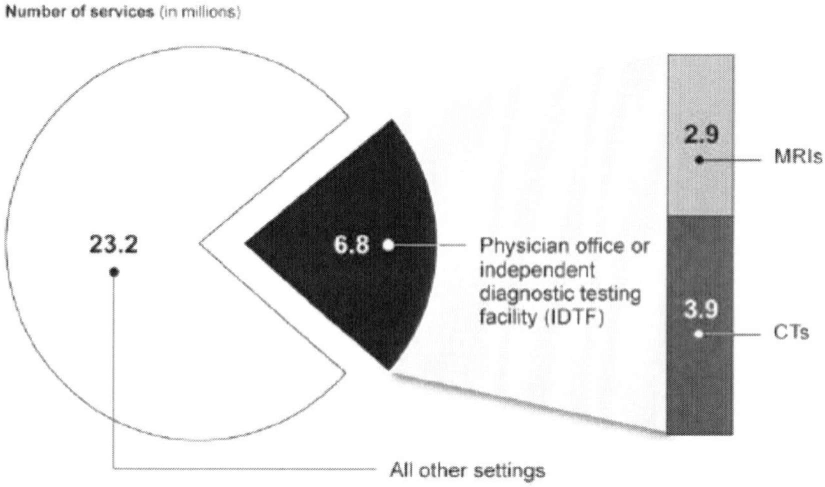

Source: GAO analysis of Medicare data.

Figure 1. Distribution of Advanced Imaging Services by Modality and Setting, 2010.

Select Implemented or Proposed Policies Designed to Address Utilization or Expenditures Associated with Self-Referral of Advanced Imaging Services

Numerous policies have been implemented or proposed by CMS, MedPAC, or other researchers that are designed to limit self-referral or reduce inappropriate utilization of advanced imaging services. These policies can affect self-referral or advanced imaging utilization through various means such as prohibiting different types of physician self-referral, informing beneficiaries of physician self-referral, mandating accreditation of staff performing MRI and CT services, improving payment accuracy, reducing payments for self-referred services, and ensuring services are clinically appropriate. One type of physician self-referral arrangement that CMS has prohibited is "per-click" self-referral arrangements where, for instance, a physician leases an imaging machine to a hospital, refers patients for imaging services, and then is paid on a per-service basis by the hospital. CMS has also solicited comments on prohibiting self-referral of diagnostic tests provided as an ancillary service in a physician's office that are not usually provided during an office visit, because a key rationale for permitting self-referral of such services is that receiving a diagnostic service during the same office visit when a physician orders a test is convenient for beneficiaries. MedPAC, in its June 2010 report to Congress, noted that MRI and CT services were performed on the same day as an office visit less than a quarter of the time, with only 8.4 percent of MRI services of the brain being performed on the same day as an office visit.[22] Appendix II lists a select number of such policies in addition to these two policies that have been implemented or put forth by CMS, MedPAC, and other researchers.

Self-Referred MRI and CT Services and Expenditures Grew Overall, While NonSelf-Referred Services and Expenditures Grew Slower or Decreased

From 2004 through 2010, the number of self-referred MRI and CT services performed in a provider's office and non-self-referred MRI and CT services performed in a provider's office or IDTF increased, with the larger increase for self-referred services. Similarly, expenditures for self-referred advanced imaging services also increased over this period, and this increase was larger than the changes in expenditures for advanced imaging services that were not self-referred. Over the period we reviewed, the share of advanced imaging services that were self-referred also increased overall and across all provider specialties we examined.

Number of Self-Referred and Non-Self-Referred MRI and CT Services Increased Overall from 2004 to 2010, with the Larger Increase among Self-Referred Services

While the number of self-referred MRI services performed in a provider's office and non-self-referred MRI services performed in a provider's office or IDTF both increased from 2004 through 2010, a significantly larger increase occurred among the self-referred services.[23] Specifically, the number of self-referred MRI services increased from about 380,000 services in 2004 to about 700,000 services in 2010—an increase of more than 80 percent (see fig 2). In contrast, the number of non-self-referred MRI services grew about 12 percent over the same time period, from about 1.97 million services in 2004 to about 2.21 million services in 2010. Despite an overall increase during this time, both self-referred and nonself-referred services declined at some point during the years of our study. However, the number of self-referred services grew faster in the earlier years and declined less in the later years than the number of nonself-referred services.

Similar to MRI services, the number of self-referred and non-self-referred CT services both increased from 2004 through 2010, with a considerably larger increase occurring in self-referred services. Specifically, the number of self-referred CT services more than doubled from 2004 through 2010, growing from about 700,000 services to about 1.45 million services (see figure 3). In contrast, the number of non-self-referred CT services increased about 30 percent during these years, from about 1.90 million services to about 2.48 million services. Although the number of both self-referred and non-self-referred CT services increased over the period of our study, the number of non-self-referred CT services decreased from 2009 through 2010.

The number of self-referred advanced imaging services increased from 2004 through 2010, even after accounting for change in the number of Medicare FFS beneficiaries. Specifically, the number of self-referred MRI services per 1,000 Medicare FFS beneficiaries grew from 10.8 in 2004 to 20.0 in 2010—an increase of about 85 percent. Similarly, the number of self-referred CT services per 1,000 Medicare FFS beneficiaries more than doubled, growing from about 19.6 in 2004 to 41.2 in 2010.

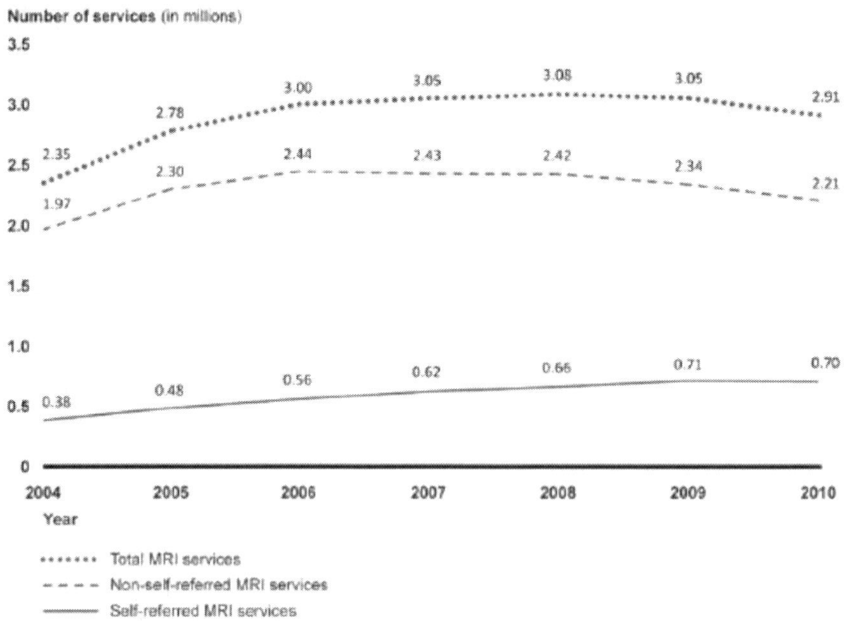

Source: GAO analysis of Medicare data.

Note: Results include services performed in a physician office or IDTF. Services performed in other settings, such as hospital outpatient departments, are not included.

Figure 2. Number of Self-Referred and Non-Self-Referred MRI Services, 2004-2010.

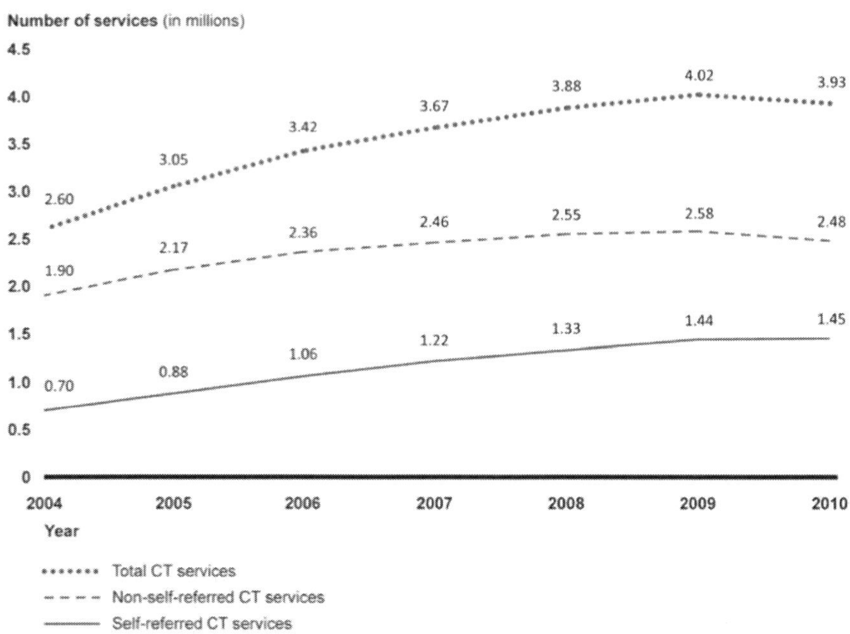

Source: GAO analysis of Medicare data.

Note: Results include services performed in a physician office or IDTF. Services performed in other settings, such as hospital outpatient departments, are not included.

Figure 3. Number of Self-Referred and Non-Self-Referred CT Services, 2004-2010.

Self-Referred MRI and CT Expenditures Grew More Than Non-Self-Referred Expenditures Overall with Non-Self-Referred MRI Expenditures Declining

Expenditures for self-referred MRI services grew overall from 2004 through 2010, while expenditures for non-self-referred MRI services declined. Specifically, self-referred MRI expenditures grew about 55 percent during the time of our review, from approximately $239 million in 2004 to about $370 million in 2010 (see figure 4).

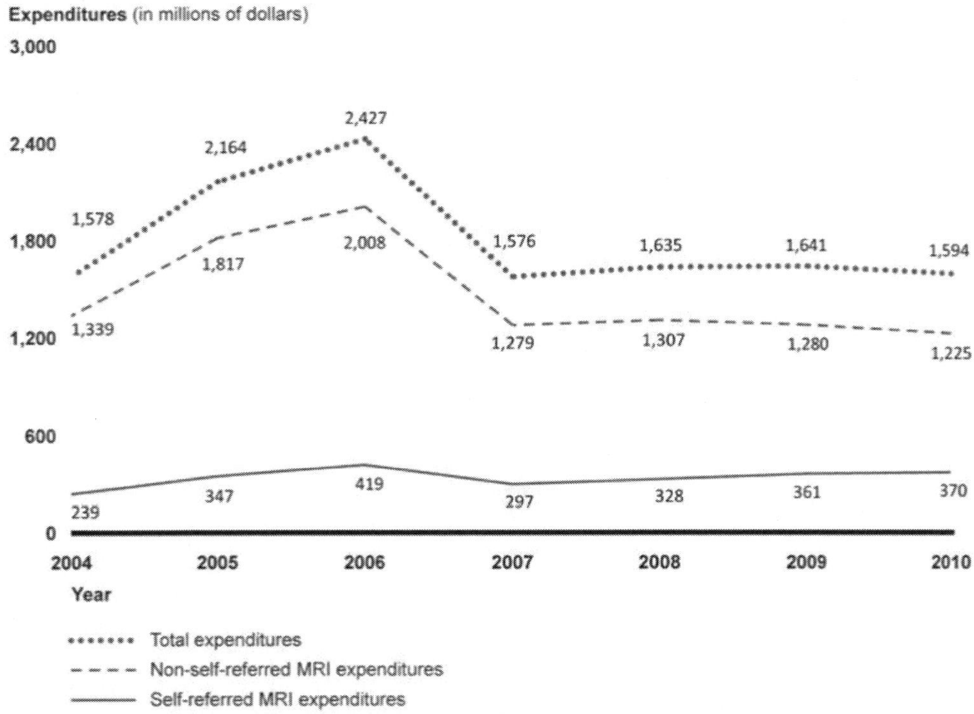

Source: GAO analysis of Medicare data.

Note: Expenditures include those services we could determine were performed in a physician office or IDTF setting. This included global claims where the performance and interpretation of the advanced imaging service were billed together—and claims where the performance of the advanced imaging service was billed separately from the interpretation of the image. We excluded expenditures for claims where the interpretation of the exam was billed separately because this service may have been performed in another setting, such as a hospital outpatient department.

Figure 4. Self-Referred and Non-Self-Referred MRI Expenditures, 2004-2010.

In contrast, expenditures for non-self-referred MRI services decreased about 8.5 percent during the same period. Expenditures for both self-referred and non-self-referred MRI services increased rapidly from 2004 through 2006, then decreased sharply in 2007. These declines in 2007 corresponded with the first year of implementation of a DRA provision that reduced fees for certain advanced imaging services.[24] Since the declines in 2007, expenditures for non-self-referred MRI services have declined further while self-referred expenditures have increased.

Relative to 2004, expenditures for both self-referred and non-self-referred CT services have grown through 2010, but the increase was larger for self-referred CT services (see figure 5).

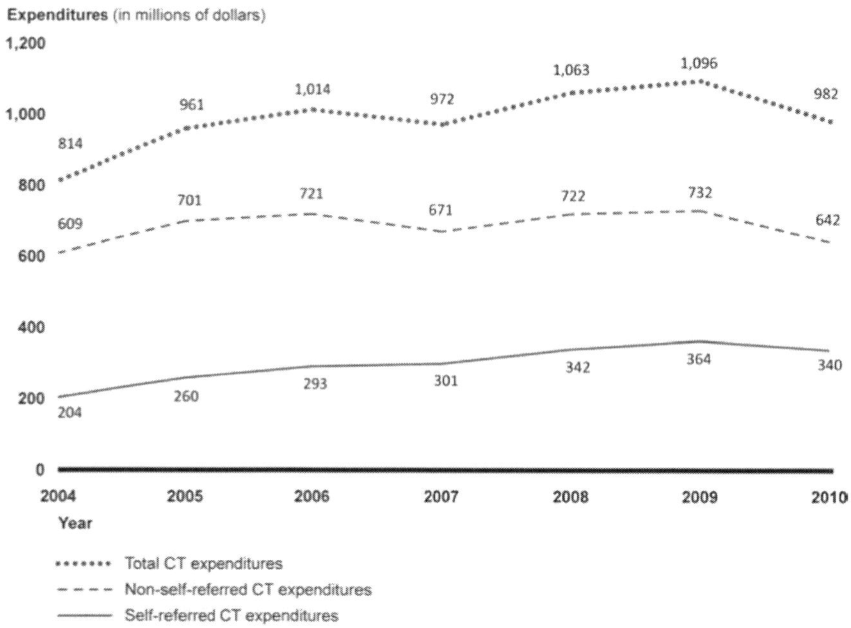

Source: GAO analysis of Medicare data.

Note: Expenditures include those services we could determine were performed in a physician office or IDTF setting. This included global claims where the performance and interpretation of the advanced imaging service were billed together—and claims where the performance of the advanced imaging service was billed separately from the interpretation of the image. We excluded expenditures for claims where the interpretation of the exam was billed separately because this service may have been performed in another setting, such as a hospital outpatient department.

Figure 5. Self-Referred and Non-Self-Referred CT Expenditures, 2004-2010.

Specifically, expenditures for self-referred CT services increased from $204 million in 2004 to about $340 million in 2010, an increase of about 67 percent.

In contrast, expenditures for non-self-referred CT services increased from about $609 million in 2004 to about $642 million in 2010, an increase of about 5 percent.

Share of Self-Referred MRI and CT Services Increased Overall and across All Major Referring Provider Specialties

Because the self-referred advanced imaging services grew at a greater rate than non-self-referred services from 2004 through 2010, the proportion of MRI and CT services that were self-referred increased during that time period. Specifically, the proportion of MRI services that were self-referred increased from 16.3 percent in 2004 to 24. 2 percent in 2010. Similarly, the proportion of CT services that were self-referred grew from 26.8 percent in 2004 to 37.0 percent in 2010.

Consistent with the overall trend, the proportion of MRI and CT services that were self-referred increased from 2004 through 2010 for all provider specialties that we studied.[25]

For further information on self-referral rates across provider specialties, see appendix III.

SELF-REFERRING PROVIDERS REFERRED SUBSTANTIALLY MORE ADVANCED IMAGING SERVICES ON AVERAGE THAN DID OTHER PROVIDERS

We found that, in 2010, providers that self-referred beneficiaries for MRI and CT services referred substantially more of those services than did providers who did not self-refer these services, even after we accounted for differences in practice size, specialty, geography, and patient characteristics. We also found that the year after providers purchased MRI or CT equipment, leased MRI or CT equipment, or joined a group practice that self-referred, they increased the number of services they referred when compared with providers that did not begin to self-refer advanced imaging services.

Self-Referring Providers Referred Substantially More MRI and CT Services Than Other Providers, Regardless of Practice or Patient Characteristics

In 2010, self-referring providers referred substantially more advanced imaging services than providers who did not self-refer such services that year.[26] Specifically, providers that self-referred at least one beneficiary for an MRI service in 2010 averaged 36.4 MRI referrals, compared with an average of 14.4 MRI referrals for non-self-referrers. Similarly, providers that self-referred at least one beneficiary for a CT service in 2010 averaged 73.2 CT referrals, or 2.3 times as many as the 32.3 CT referrals averaged by non-self-referring providers. About 10 percent of all MRI and CT services referred by self-referring providers in 2010 were ordered, performed, and interpreted by the same provider.

Certain efficiencies may be gained when the same provider orders, performs, and interprets an advanced imaging service, such as reviewing a patient's clinical history only once. CMS has taken steps to ensure that fees for services paid under the physician fee schedule take into account efficiencies that resulted from how the services are provided, and we recently recommended that CMS expand these efforts.[27]

Differences in advanced imaging referrals between self-referring and nonself-referring providers persisted after accounting for differences in practice size, specialty, geography, or patient characteristics.

Practice Size

Self-referring providers referred more MRI and CT services than did nonself-referring providers, regardless of differences in practice size. In general, self-referring providers tend to work in practices with a larger number of Medicare beneficiaries.

However, in 2010, self-referring providers referred more MRI and CT services than non-self-referring providers regardless of practice size, and the difference in number of services referred generally increased as provider size increased (see table 1). For example, self-referring providers that had 50 or fewer patients referred 1.8 times as many MRI services as did non-self-referring providers. In comparison, self-referring providers with 500 or more patients referred 2.4 times as many MRI services as non-self-referring providers did.

Table 1. Average Number of MRI and CT Services Referred by Non-Self-Referring and Self-Referring Providers, 2010

	MRI services			CT services		
Number of unique Medicare FFS beneficiaries[a]	Non-self-referring	Self-referring	Relative rate of self-referring providers[b]	Non-self-referring	Self-referring	Relative rate of self-referring providers[b]
1 to 50	3.2	5.7	1.8	5.2	7.1	1.4
51 to 100	7.2	12.3	1.7	13.7	19.0	1.4
101 to 250	13.0	24.0	1.8	26.7	40.8	1.5
251 to 500	20.4	42.8	2.1	48.7	78.8	1.6
>500	29.7	71.1	2.4	89.9	151.0	1.7

Source: GAO analysis of Medicare data.

Notes: Providers were considered to be self-referring if they self-referred beneficiaries for at least one service. Providers with a specialty of radiology or independent diagnostic testing facility (IDTF) were removed from this analysis because they should not be able to self-refer services. Additionally, because emergency medicine providers generally did not practice in provider offices, they were removed from our analysis. Of the 419,884 providers that referred at least one beneficiary for an MRI service in 2010, 35,950 were self-referring and 383,934 were non-self-referring. Of the 477,547 providers that referred at least one beneficiary for a CT service in 2010, 39,913 were self-referring and 437,634 were non-self-referring.

[a]The number of unique Medicare FFS beneficiaries refers to the number of unique beneficiaries that received at least one service from a provider.

[b]The relative rate of self-referring providers refers to the factor by which the average number of services referred by self-referring providers is greater than the average number of services referred by non-self-referring providers. For example, if the relative rate of self-referring providers is equal to 3, it would mean that, on average, self-referrers refer 3 times as many advanced imaging services as do non-self-referrers.

Specialty

Self-referring providers generally referred more MRI and CT services than did non-self-referring providers, regardless of differences in specialties. Self-referring providers were more likely than non-self-referring providers to belong to specialties that had a greater-than-average number of referrals per physician for advanced imaging services in 2010.

However, for the 7 specialties that had at least 1,000 providers that self-referred beneficiaries for MRI services, self-referring providers generally averaged more referrals for MRI services than did non-self-referring providers, regardless of practice size.[28]

Similarly, self-referring providers in 9 of the 13 specialties that had at least 1,000 self-referring CT providers generally referred more beneficiaries for CT services than non-self-referring providers, regardless of practice size.[29]

Table 2. Average Number of MRI and CT Services Referred by Non-Self-Referring and Self-Referring Providers in Urban and Rural Locations, 2010

Geographic designation			MRI services			CT services	
	Number of unique Medicare FFS beneficiaries[a]	Non-self-referring	Self-referring	Relative rate of self-referring providers[b]	Non-self-referring	Self-referring	Relative rate of self-referring providers[b]
Urban	1 to 50	3.3	5.8	1.8	5.4	7.3	1.4
	51 to 100	7.5	12.4	1.7	14.2	19.4	1.4
	101 to 250	13.5	24.4	1.8	27.2	41.9	1.5
	251 to 500	20.8	43.9	2.1	48.2	80.8	1.7
	>500	29.5	72.1	2.4	86.5	151.5	1.8
Rural	1 to 50	2.8	4.7	1.7	4.3	5.2	1.2
	51 to 100	5.7	10.2	1.8	10.4	12.7	1.2
	101 to 250	10.5	20.1	1.9	23.8	30.3	1.3
	251 to 500	19.0	34.6	1.8	51.3	64.7	1.3
	>500	30.5	65.4	2.1	102.8	147.8	1.4

Source: GAO analysis of Medicare data.

Notes: Providers were considered to be self-referring if they self-referred beneficiaries for at least one service. Providers with a specialty of radiology or independent diagnostic testing facility (IDTF) were removed from this analysis because they should not be able to self-refer services. Additionally, because emergency medicine providers generally did not practice in provider offices, they were removed from our analysis. Of the 419,884 providers that referred at least one beneficiary for an MRI service in 2010, 35,950 were self-referring and 383,934 were non-self-referring. Of the 477,547 providers that referred at least one beneficiary for a CT service in 2010, 39,913 were self-referring and 437,634 were non-self-referring.

[a]The number of unique Medicare FFS beneficiaries refers to the number of unique beneficiaries that received at least one service from a provider.

[b]The relative rate of self-referring providers refers to the factor by which the average number of services referred by self-referring providers is greater than the average number of services referred by non-self-referring providers. For example, if the relative rate of self-referring providers is equal to 3, it would mean that, on average, self-referrers refer 3 times as many advanced imaging services as do non-self-referrers.

Geography

Self-referring providers referred more MRI and CT services than non-selfreferring providers, regardless of differences in geography. Providers that self-referred MRI services averaged 36.3 MRI referrals and 37.3 MRI referrals in urban and rural locations, respectively.

In comparison, nonself-referring providers averaged 14.3 MRI referrals in urban locations and 15.2 MRI referrals in rural locations. Providers that self-referred beneficiaries for CT services averaged 72.7 referrals in urban locations and 77.2 referrals in rural locations, while non-self-referring providers averaged 31.1 CT referrals in urban locations and 40.7 referrals in rural locations.

We found that differences in the number of MRI and CT referrals made by self-referring and non-self-referring providers persisted when accounting for provider size along with geography (see table 2).

Patient Characteristics

Self-referring providers referred more MRI and CT services than non-selfreferring providers, in spite of similarities in patient characteristics. Specifically, the patient populations of self-referring and non-self-referring MRI and CT providers were similar in terms of most patient characteristics, with self-referring providers having slightly healthier patients than non-self-referring providers, as indicated by their lower average risk score (see table 3). If self-referring providers had patients that were older or sicker, it could have explained why self-referring providers referred their patients for more services than non-self-referring providers.

Providers' Referrals for MRI and CT Services Substantially Increased the Year after They Began to Self-Refer

Our analysis indicated that providers' referrals for MRI and CT services substantially increased the year after they began to self-refer. In our analysis, we compared the number of MRI and CT referrals for switchers—those providers that did not self-refer in 2007 or 2008 but did self-refer in 2009 and 2010—to providers that did not change their self-referral status during the same time period. Providers could self-refer by purchasing imaging equipment, leasing equipment, or joining a group practice that already self-referred. Overall, the switcher group of providers who began self-referring in 2009 increased the average number of MRI and CT referrals they made by about 67 percent in 2010 compared to the average in 2008. In the case of MRIs, the average number of referrals switchers made for MRI services increased from 25.1 in 2008 to 42.0 in 2010. In contrast, the average number of MRI and CT referrals declined for providers that did not self-refer and providers who self-referred from 2008 through 2010. This comparison suggests that the increase in the average number of referrals for switchers from 2008 to 2010 was not due to a general increase in the use of imaging services among all providers. (See table 4.)

The increase in MRI and CT referrals for providers that began self-referring in 2009 cannot be explained exclusively by factors such as providers joining practices with higher patient volumes, different patient populations, or different practice cultures. Specifically, providers that remained in the same practice from 2007 through 2010, but began self-referring in 2009, also had a bigger increase in the number of MRI and CT referrals than did providers that did not change their self-referral status.[30] Providers that remained in the same practice from 2008 through 2010, but began self-referring in 2009 had a 21.0 percent increase in MRI referrals and a 14.4 percent increase in CT referrals.

Table 3. Patient Characteristics of Non-Self-Referring and Self-Referring MRI and CT Providers, 2010

Patient characteristics, average	MRI services		CT services	
	Non-self-referring	Self-referring	Non-self-referring	Self-referring
Average age (years)	70	71	70	71
Percent female	59	60	59	57
Average risk score[a]	1.53	1.40	1.57	1.44

Source: GAO analysis of Medicare data.

[a]A beneficiary's risk score is a proxy for health status and is equivalent to the ratio of expected health care expenditures for that beneficiary under Medicare FFS relative to the average health care expenditures for all Medicare FFS beneficiaries. For example, a beneficiary with a risk score of 1.05 would have expected expenditures that were 5 percent higher than an average Medicare FFS beneficiary. The risk scores presented are normalized using the FFS normalization factor of 1.041 that CMS used to normalize risk scores in 2010. Normalization keeps the average Medicare FFS risk score constant at 1.0 over time.

Table 4. Change in Average Number of MRI and CT Services Referred, 2008 and 2010

Provider referral type	MRI Services				CT Services			
	Number of providers	Average 2008 referred MRI services	Average 2010 referred MRI services	Percentage change, 2008 to 2010	Number of providers	Average 2008 referred CT services	Average 2010 referred CT services	Percentage change, 2008 to 2010
Switchers	2,803	25.1	42.0	67.3	3,329	56.3	93.9	66.7
Non-self-referrers	199,102	20.6	19.2	-6.8	241,097	59.1	58.1	-1.7
Self-referrers	17,753	47.0	45.4	-3.4	19,756	89.6	87.3	-2.6

Source: GAO analysis of Medicare data.

Note: We define switchers as those providers that did not self-refer in 2007 or 2008, but did self-refer in 2009 and 2010.

HIGHER USE OF ADVANCED IMAGING SERVICES BY SELF-REFERRING PROVIDERS RESULTS IN SUBSTANTIAL COSTS TO MEDICARE

On the basis of our estimates, Medicare spent about $109 million more in 2010 than the program would have if self-referring providers referred advanced imaging services at the same rate as non-self-referring providers of the same specialty and provider size (see figure 6). This additional spending can be attributed to the fact that self-referring providers referred over 400,000 more MRI and CT services in 2010 than if they had referred at the same rate as non-self-referring providers of the same size and specialty. Specifically, we estimate there were 143,303 additional referrals for MRI services and 283,725 additional referrals for CT services.

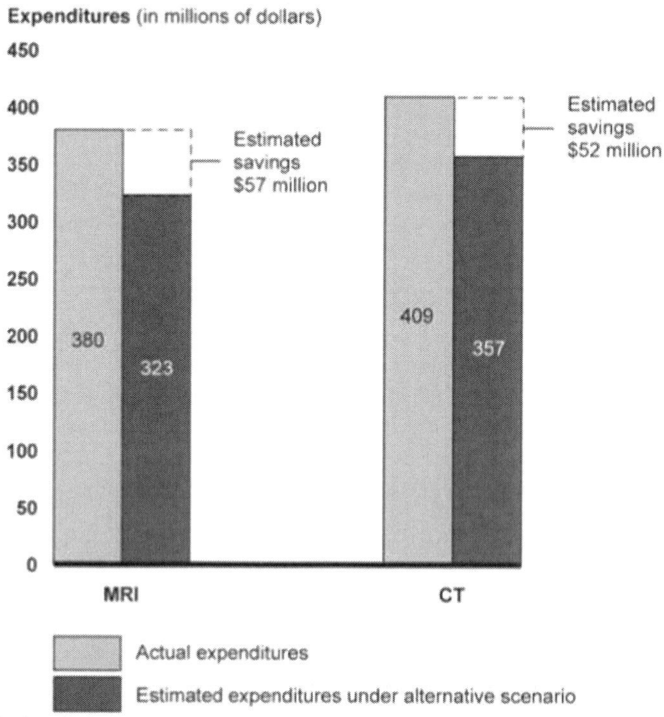

Source: GAO analysis of Medicare data.

Note: We included imaging expenditures for those specialties that had at least 1,000 self-referring providers. Overall, specialties that met these criteria referred approximately 66 percent of self-referred MRI services and approximately 81 percent of self-referred CT services. Under the alternative scenario, we calculated expenditures for services as if self-referring providers referred MRI and CT services at the same rate as non-self-referring providers of the same specialty and practice size in 2010.

Figure 6. Potential Savings under Alternative Scenario for Self-Referring Providers, 2010.

The additional Medicare imaging expenditures attributed to self-referring providers is likely higher than $109 million in 2010.[31] This is because a significant portion of self-referring providers are not included in this estimate. Specifically, we limited our analysis to those specialties that had at least 1,000 self-referring providers. Approximately 34 percent of the providers who self-referred beneficiaries for MRI services and 19 percent of the providers who self-referred beneficiaries for CT services belonged to a specialty other than those that met the 1,000 self-referring providers criteria.

CONCLUSION

Advanced imaging services can help in the early detection and aid in the treatment of certain diseases, resulting in less-invasive treatments and improved patient outcomes. The ability of providers to self-refer beneficiaries for these services can, for example, improve coordination of care and help ensure convenient access to these services among beneficiaries. However, our review indicates that some factor or factors other than the health status of patients, provider practice size or specialty, or geographic location (i.e., rural or urban) helped drive the higher advanced imaging referral rates among self-referring providers compared to non-self-referring providers.

We found that providers who began to self-refer advanced imaging services—after purchasing or leasing imaging equipment or joining practices that self-referred—substantially increased their referrals for MRI and CT services relative to other providers. This suggests that financial incentives for self-referring providers may be a major factor driving the increase in referrals.

These financial incentives likely help explain why, in 2010, providers who self-referred made 400,000 more referrals for advanced imaging services than they would have if they were not self-referring. These additional referrals cost CMS more than $100 million in 2010 alone. To the extent that these additional referrals are unnecessary, they pose an unacceptable risk for beneficiaries, particularly in the case of CT services, which involve the use of ionizing radiation.

Given the challenges to the long-range fiscal sustainability of Medicare, it is imperative that CMS develop policies to address the effect of self-referral on the utilization of and expenditures for advanced imaging services. CMS first needs to improve its ability to identify services that are self-referred.

Claims do not include an indicator or "flag" that identifies whether services are self-referred or non-self-referred, and CMS does not currently have a method for easily identifying such services. A systematic method for identifying self-referred advanced imaging services would give CMS the ongoing ability to determine the extent to which these services are self-referred and help the agency identify those services that may be inappropriate, unnecessary, or potentially harmful to beneficiaries. Including a self-referral flag on Medicare Part B claims submitted by providers who bill for advanced imaging services is likely the easiest and most cost-effective approach. Second, we found that about 10 percent of advanced imaging services referred by self-referring physicians in 2010 were also performed and interpreted by the same physician.

Certain efficiencies may be gained when the same provider orders, performs, and interprets an advanced imaging service, such as reviewing a patient's clinical history only once. MedPAC recommended in 2011 that CMS should reduce its payments for advanced imaging services in which the same provider refers and performs the service, to account for efficiencies that are realized in these circumstances.

This is consistent with previous efforts by CMS to reduce fees for services paid under the physician fee schedule when efficiencies are realized and with our previous recommendation that CMS expand these efforts.

Third, if CMS were able to easily identify self-referred services, the agency may be better positioned to implement an approach that ensures the appropriateness of advanced imaging services that Medicare beneficiaries receive—beyond examining the feasibility of such methods, as we recommended in our 2008 report. Approaches for managing advanced imaging utilization could be "front-end" or used before CMS issues payment, such as prior authorization.

CMS could also explore back-end approaches used after CMS issues payment, such as targeted audits of self-referring providers that refer a high volume of services.

Recommendations for Executive Action

In order to improve CMS's ability to identify self-referred advanced imaging services and help CMS address the increases in these services, we recommend that the Administrator of CMS take the following three actions:

1. Insert a self-referral flag on its Medicare Part B claims form and require providers to indicate whether the advanced imaging services for which a provider bills Medicare are self-referred or not.
2. Determine and implement a payment reduction for self-referred advanced imaging services to recognize efficiencies when the same provider refers and performs a service.
3. Determine and implement an approach to ensure the appropriateness of advanced imaging services referred by self-referring providers.

Agency Comments and Our Evaluation

HHS reviewed a draft of this report and provided written comments. In its comments, HHS stated that it would consider one of our recommendations but did not concur with our other two recommendations. HHS did not comment on our findings that self-referring providers referred substantially more advanced imaging services than non-self-referring providers or our conclusion that financial incentives for self-referring providers may be a major factor driving the increase in referrals for advanced imaging services.

HHS noted that it would consider our recommendation that CMS determine and implement an approach to ensure the appropriateness of advanced imaging services referred by self-referring providers. According to HHS, CMS would consider this recommendation when refining its medical review strategy for advanced imaging services. HHS also indicated that CMS does not have statutory authority to implement some of the approaches discussed in the report. We are pleased that CMS plans to consider this recommendation and note that we did not identify a specific approach, having identified several examples in our report of both front-end and back-end approaches to managing utilization of advanced imaging services. As we reported, CMS could explore back-end approaches used after CMS issues payment, such as targeted audits of self-referring providers. CMS could also explore other approaches the agency determines are within its statutory authority. Further, if deemed necessary, CMS could seek legislative authority to implement promising approaches to managing advanced imaging utilization.

HHS did not concur with our recommendation that CMS insert a self-referral flag on its Medicare Part B claims and require providers to indicate whether the advanced imaging services for which a provider bills Medicare are self-referred or not. According to HHS, CMS believes that a new checkbox on the claim form identifying self-referral would be complex to administer and providers may not characterize referrals accurately. CMS believes that other payment reforms, such as paying networks of providers, hospitals, or other entities that share responsibility for providing care to patients, would better address overutilization. We continue to believe that including an indicator or flag on the claims would likely be the easiest and most cost-effective approach to improve CMS's ability to identify self-referred advanced imaging services. We do not suggest, nor did we intend, that CMS use the self-referral flag or indicator we recommended to determine compliance with the physician self-referral law. Without a self-referral flag or indicator, CMS will not be able to monitor trends in utilization and expenditures associated with physician self-referral without considerable time and effort. Further, a self-referral flag does not have to be a "checkbox" on the claim and could be a modifier, similar to other modifiers that CMS uses to characterize claims. In addition, HHS did not provide reasons to support CMS's contention that such a flag would be complex to administer.

HHS also did not concur with our recommendation that CMS determine and implement a payment reduction for self-referred advanced imaging services to recognize efficiencies when the same provider refers and performs a service. According to HHS, CMS's multiple procedure payment reduction already captures efficiencies inherent in providing multiple advanced imaging services by the same physician or group practice during the same session. CMS also noted that a further payment reduction may reduce, but not eliminate, the underlying financial incentive to self-refer advanced imaging services and may cause providers to refer more services, in an effort to maintain their income. CMS also noted that providers in a group practice could easily avoid this reduction by having one physician order the service while another furnishes the service. According to HHS, CMS also questions its statutory authority to impose the payment reduction for the subset of physicians who self-refer, citing a prohibition on paying a differential by physician specialty for the same service. Our report shows that self-referring providers generally referred more MRI and CT services, regardless of differences in specialties, and CMS did not indicate how this recommendation would implicate the prohibition on paying a differential by specialty. Additionally, while HHS cites the multiple procedure payment reduction as a means to address certain efficiencies in the delivery of advanced imaging services, these are not the efficiencies targeted by our recommendation. Instead, as noted in our report, our recommended payment reduction would capture those efficiencies gained when the same provider orders and performs an advanced imaging service. Such efficiencies could be captured in a single—rather than multiple—advanced imaging service. This recommendation is also consistent with a 2011 MedPAC recommendation. As noted in our report, this payment reduction would affect about 10 percent of advanced imaging services referred by self-referring providers. As for CMS's concern about overutilization of advanced imaging services resulting from a payment reduction, CMS could help address this issue by implementing our recommendation to use a flag indicating self-referral to monitor utilization of these services.

On the basis of HHS's written response to our report, we are concerned that neither HHS nor CMS appears to recognize the need to monitor the self-referral of advanced imaging services on an ongoing basis and determine those services that may be inappropriate, unnecessary, or potentially harmful to beneficiaries. HHS did not comment on our key finding that self-referring physicians referred about two times as many advanced imaging services, on average, as providers who did not self refer. Nor did HHS comment on our estimate that these additional referrals for advanced imaging services cost CMS more than $100 million in 2010 alone. Given these findings, we continue to believe that CMS should take steps to monitor the utilization of advanced imaging services and ensure that the services for which Medicare pays are appropriate.

HHS also provided technical comments that we incorporated as appropriate.

James C. Cosgrove
Director,
Health Care

APPENDIX I: SCOPE AND METHODS

This section describes the scope and methodology used to analyze our three objectives: (1) trends in the number of and expenditures for self-referred and non-self-referred advanced imaging services from 2004 through 2010, (2) the extent to which the provision of advanced imaging services differs for providers who self-refer when compared with other providers, and (3) the implications of self-referral for Medicare spending on advanced imaging services.

For all three objectives, we used the Medicare Part B Carrier File, which contains final action Medicare Part B claims for noninstitutional providers, such as physicians. Claims can be for one or more services or for individual service components.[1] Each service or service component is identified on a claim by its Healthcare Common Procedure Coding System (HCPCS) code, which the Centers for Medicare & Medicaid Services (CMS) assigns to products, supplies, and services for billing purposes. HCPCS codes are also categorized by CMS using the Berenson-Eggers Type of Service (BETOS) categorization system, which assigns HCPCS to broad service categories.[2]

We limited our universe of services and service components for our study to those for magnetic resonance imaging (MRI) and computed tomography (CT) services. We classified MRI and CT services and service components as those with HCPCS codes included in a BETOS category where the first two digits were equal to "I2", defined as advanced imaging services. We further limited our universe to only those MRI and CT services that were considered designated health services—services for which, in the absence of an exception, a physician may not make a referral to furnish to an entity with which he has a without implicating the Stark law.[3] Annually, CMS publishes a list of designated health services as part of the physician fee schedule. We also restricted our universe to those HCPCS codes that involved the performance of an advanced imaging service, which can be billed with or separately from the interpretation of a MRI or CT imaging service. We identified 125 HCPCS codes that met these criteria.

Because there is no indicator or "flag" on the claim that identifies whether services were self-referred or non-self-referred, we developed a claims-based methodology for identifying self-referred services. Specifically, we classified services as self-referred if the provider that referred the beneficiary for a MRI or CT service and the provider that performed the MRI or CT service was identical or had a financial relationship with the same entity. We used taxpayer identification number (TIN), an identification number used by the Internal Revenue Service, to determine providers' financial relationships. The TIN could be that of the provider, the provider's employer, or another entity to which the provider reassigns payment. [4] In order to identify the associated TINs for the referring and performing providers, we created a crosswalk of the performing provider's unique physician identification number or national provider identifier (NPI) financial relationship without implicating the Stark law.[3] Annually, CMS publishes a list of designated health services as part of the physician fee schedule. We also restricted our universe to those HCPCS codes that involved the performance of an advanced imaging service, which can be billed with or separately from the interpretation of a MRI or CT imaging service. We identified 125 HCPCS codes that met these criteria.

Because there is no indicator or "flag" on the claim that identifies whether services were self-referred or non-self-referred, we developed a claims-based methodology for identifying self-referred services. Specifically, we classified services as self-referred if the provider that referred the beneficiary for a MRI or CT service and the provider that performed the MRI or CT service was identical or had a financial relationship with the same entity. We used taxpayer identification number (TIN), an identification number used by the Internal Revenue Service, to determine providers' financial relationships. The TIN could be that of the provider, the provider's employer, or another entity to which the provider reassigns payment. [4] In order to identify the associated TINs for the referring and performing providers, we created a crosswalk of the performing provider's unique physician identification number or national provider identifier (NPI) to the TIN that appeared on the claim and used that to assign TINs to the referring and performing providers.[5]

We considered global services and separately-billed TCs to be self-referred if one or more of the TINs of the referring and performing provider matched. However, we did not consider separately-billed PCs to be self-referred, even if they met the same criterion. Compared to the payment for the TC of an advanced imaging service, the payment for the PC is relatively small, and thus there is little incentive for providers to only self-refer the PC of a service. As part of developing this claims-based methodology to identify self-referred services, we interviewed officials from CMS, provider groups, and other researchers.

To describe the trends in the number of and expenditures for self-referred and non-self-referred advanced imaging services from 2004 through 2010, we used the Medicare Part B Carrier File to calculate utilization and expenditures for self-referred and non-self-referred MRI and CT services, both in aggregate and per beneficiary. We limited this portion of our analysis to global claims or claims for a separately-billed TC, which indicates that the performance of the imaging service was billed under the physician fee schedule. As a result, the universe for this portion of our analysis are those advanced imaging services performed in a provider's office or in an independent diagnostic testing facility (IDTF), which both bill for the performance of an advanced imaging service under the physician fee schedule. We focused on these settings because our previous work showed rapid growth among such services and because the financial incentive for providers to self-refer is most direct when the service is performed in a physician office. Approximately one-fifth of all advanced imaging services provided to Medicare FFS beneficiaries were performed in a physician office or IDTF. To calculate the number of Medicare beneficiaries from 2004 through 2010 needed for per beneficiary calculations, we used the Denominator File, a database that contains enrollment information for all Medicare beneficiaries enrolled in a given year. Because radiologists and IDTFs are limited in their ability to generate referrals for advanced imaging services, we removed services referred by an IDTF or radiologist.

To determine the extent to which the provision of advanced imaging services differs for providers who self-refer when compared with other providers, we first classified providers on the basis of the type of referrals they made. Specifically, we classified providers as self-referring if they self-referred at least one beneficiary for an advanced imaging service.[6] We classified providers as non-self-referring if they referred a beneficiary for an advanced imaging service, but did not self-refer any of the services. Because radiologists and providers in IDTFs predominantly perform advanced imaging services and have limited ability to refer beneficiaries for advanced imaging services, we removed those providers from our analysis. Additionally, because emergency medicine providers generally did not practice in provider offices, they were removed from our analysis. We assigned to each provider the MRI and CT service and service-components that he or she referred, including those for the performance of an imaging service and those for the interpretation of the imaging service result. If the TC and PC were billed separately for the same beneficiary, we counted these two components as one referred service. As a result, we counted all services that a provider referred, regardless of whether it was performed in a provider office, IDTF, or other setting. We then performed two separate analyses.

First, we compared the provision—that is, the number of referrals made— of MRI and CT services by self-referring providers and non-self-referring providers in 2010, after accounting for factors such as practice size (i.e., the number of Medicare beneficiaries), provider specialty, geography (i.e., urban or rural), and patient characteristics. We used the number of unique Medicare fee-for-service (FFS) beneficiaries for which providers provided services in 2010 as a proxy for practice size, which we identified using 100 percent of providers' claims from the Medicare Part B Carrier File. We defined urban settings as metropolitan statistical areas, a geographic entity defined by the Office of Management and Budget as a core urban area of 50,000 or more population. We used rural-urban commuting area codes—a Census tract-based classification scheme that utilizes the standard Bureau of Census Urbanized Area and Urban Cluster definitions in combination with work-commuting information to characterize all of the nation's Census tracts regarding their rural and urban status—to identify providers as practicing in metropolitan statistical areas.[7] We considered all other settings to be rural. We identified providers' specialties on the basis of the specialties listed on the claims. These specialty codes include physician specialties, such as cardiology and hematology/oncology, and nonphysician provider types, such as nurse practitioners and physician assistants. We also examined the extent to which the characteristics of the patient populations served by self-referring and non-self-referring providers differed. We used CMS's risk score file to identify average risk score, which serves as a proxy for beneficiary health status. Information on additional patient characteristics, such as age and sex, came from the Medicare Part B Carrier File claims. To calculate the percentage of advanced imaging services referred by self-referring providers that were referred, performed, and interpreted by the same provider, we summed global advanced imaging claims where the referring and performing provider were the same and claims where the TC and PC were referred and performed separately for the same beneficiary by the same provider. We then divided the total by the number MRI and CT services referred by self-referring providers.

Second, we determined the extent to which the number of MRI and CT referrals made by providers changed after they began to self-refer. Specifically, we identified a group of providers that began to self-refer advanced imaging services in 2009. [8] We refer to this group of providers as "switchers" because it represents providers that did not self-refer in 2007 or 2008, but did self-refer in 2009 and 2010. We then calculated the change in the number of MRI or CT referrals made from 2008 (i.e., the year before the switchers began self-referring) to 2010 (i.e., the year after they began self-referring). We compared the change in the number of referrals made by these providers to the change in the number of referrals made over the same time period by providers who did not change whether or not they self-referred advanced imaging services. Specifically, we compared the change in the number of referrals made by switchers to those made by (1) self-referring providers—providers that self-referred in years 2007 through 2010, and (2) non-self-referring providers—providers that did not self-refer in years 2007 through 2010. For each provider, we also identified the most common TIN to which they referred MRI or CT services. If the TIN was the same for all 4 years, we assumed that they remained part of the same practice for all 4 years. We calculated the number of referrals in 2008 and 2010 separately for providers that met this criterion.

To determine the implications of self-referral for Medicare spending on advanced imaging services, we summed the number of and expenditures for all MRI and CT services performed in 2010 by providers of those specialties with at least 1,000 self-referring providers. We then created an alternative scenario in which self-referring providers referred the same number of services as non-self-referring providers of the same provider size and specialty and calculated how this affected expenditures. To do this, we calculated the number of advanced imaging services non-selfreferring providers referred per unique Medicare FFS beneficiary for each specialty and practice size. We then multiplied the referral rate times the number of patients seen by self-referring providers of the same practice size and specialty, representing the number of services self-referring providers would have referred if they referred at the non-self-referring rate. To calculate the cost of additional services to Medicare, we multiplied the difference between the self-referred services and the number of services they would have referred if they referred at the same rate as non-self-referring providers by the average expenditures for a MRI or CT service.

We took several steps to ensure that the data used to produce this report were sufficiently reliable. Specifically, we assessed the reliability of the CMS data we used by interviewing officials responsible for overseeing these data sources, reviewing relevant documentation, and examining the data for obvious errors. We determined that the data were sufficiently reliable for the purposes of our study.

We conducted this performance audit from May 2010 through September 2012 in accordance with generally accepted government auditing standards. Those standards require that we plan and perform the audit to obtain sufficient, appropriate evidence to provide a reasonable basis for our findings and conclusions based on our audit objectives. We believe that the evidence obtained provides a reasonable basis for our findings and conclusions based on our audit objectives.

APPENDIX II: SELECT IMPLEMENTED OR PROPOSED POLICIES DESIGNED TO ADDRESS SELF-REFERRAL OR THE UTILIZATION OF ADVANCED IMAGING SERVICES

Policy approach	Description and examples of policies
Informing Beneficiaries of Physician Self-Referral	Effective January 1, 2011, the Patient Protection and Affordable Care Act of 2010 (PPACA) requires physicians who self-refer MRI, CT, or positron emission tomography services under certain circumstances to inform their patients that they may obtain these services from another provider and provide their patients with a list of alternative providers in their area.[a] The effect of this requirement on physician self-referral is unclear. The American College of Radiology reports that multiple states had similar requirements in place before the implementation of PPACA.[b]

Appendix II. (Continued)

Policy approach	Description and examples of policies
Mandating Accreditation of Staff Performing MRI and CT Services	In 2008, the Centers for Medicare and Medicaid (CMS) proposed, but did not adopt, a requirement that provider office-based imaging practices enroll as independent diagnostic testing facilities (IDTF).[c] However, the Medicare Improvements for Patients and Providers Act of 2008 requires physicians and other providers to be accredited by a CMS-approved national accreditation organization by January 1, 2012,
	in order to continue to furnish the technical component of services such as MRI and CT services.[d] While the intent of this requirement was to improve quality of care, this policy could reduce the number of providers who self-refer if they fail to gain accreditation. However, this policy's actual effect on self-referral is unclear.
Improving Payment Accuracy	The Medicare Payment Advisory Commission (MedPAC) has noted that improving the payment accuracy of services could reduce the incentive to self-refer those services by making them less financially beneficial.[e] Consistent with our previous recommendations, payment rates for MRI and CT services have been reduced several times over the last few years to reflect efficiencies that occur when the same provider performs multiple services on the same patient on the same day.[f,g]
Reducing Payments for Physician Self-Referred Services Ensuring Services are Clinically Appropriate	In its June 2010 report, MedPAC noted that reducing payments for physician self-referred services could limit Medicare expenditures when self-referral occurs and reduce the incentive to self-refer by making it less financially beneficial.[h] One option put forth in the report is reducing payments for certain self-referred services by an amount equal to the percent expenditures increase due to self-referral. Another option discussed is reducing the payment for self-referred services when they include activities already performed by self-referring physicians, such as reviewing the medical history of a beneficiary.
Ensuring Services are Clinically Appropriate	In addition to a similar recommendation from MedPAC, we have recommended CMS consider expanding its front-end management capabilities, such as prior authorization—an approach whereby providers must seek some sort of approval before ordering an advanced imaging service.[i,j] Such policies could limit the increased utilization associated with self-referral by ensuring that self-referred services are clinically appropriate. One researcher suggested expanding postpayment reviews by making imaging a subject for medical review by recovery audit contractors.[k,l]
Prohibiting Different Types of Physician Self-Referral	CMS has prohibited different types of physician self-referral that the agency deemed particularly susceptible to abuse. Effective October 1, 2009, CMS prohibits "per-click" self-referral arrangements where, for instance, a physician leases an imaging machine to a hospital, refers patients to that hospital in order to receive imaging services, and then is paid on a per service basis by the hospital.[m] In 2008, CMS considered but did not prohibit "block time" self-referral arrangements where, for instance, a physician leases a block of time on a facility's MRI or CT machine, refers his or her patients to receive services on the facility's machine, and then bills for the services.[n] CMS has also solicited comments on a prohibition against physician self-referral for diagnostic tests provided in physician offices when those tests are not needed at the time of a patient's office visit in order to assist the physician in determining an appropriate diagnosis or plan of treatment.[o] MedPAC has found that MRI and CT services are performed on the same day as an office visit less than a quarter of the time, with only 8.4 percent of MRIs of the brain being performed on the same day as an office visit.[p] Another policy, discussed in MedPAC's June 2010 report, that would limit physician

Policy approach	Description and examples of policies
	selfreferral is restricting certain types of self-referral to only those practices that are clinically integrated. Maryland prohibits providers from making self-referrals for certain MRI and CT services.[q]

Source: GAO analysis of select self-referral regulations and proposals.

[a] Pub. L. No. 11-148, § 6003, 124 Stat. 199, 697.

[b] American College of Radiology, State-by-State Comparison of Physician Self-Referral Laws, accessed July 26, 2010.

[c] Medicare Program; Revisions to Payment Policies Under the Physician Fee Schedule and Other Revisions to Part B for CY 2009, 73 Fed. Reg. 38502, 28533 (July 7, 2008).

[d] Pub. L. No. 110-275, §135(a), 122 Stat. 2494, 2532.

[e] See Medicare Payment Advisory Commission, Report to Congress: Aligning Incentives in Medicare (Washington, D.C.: June 2010).

[f] See GAO, Medicare Physician Payments: Fees Could Better Reflect Efficiencies Achieved When Services Are Provided Together, GAO-09-647 (Washington, D.C.: July 31, 2009).

[g] For instance, in 2006, CMS began reducing the payment for the technical component of the lower-priced imaging service by 25 percent when multiple services are performed on contiguous body parts during the same session. See Medicare Program: Revisions to Payment Policies Under the Physician Fee Schedule for Calendar Year 2006, 70 Fed. Reg. 70116 (Nov. 21, 2005). PPACA increased the payment reduction from 25 percent to 50 percent beginning July 1, 2010. Pub. L. No. 111-148, §3135(b), 124 Stat. 119, 437. CMS also expanded this policy beginning January 1, 2012 by reducing payments for the lower-priced professional component of advanced imaging services by 25 percent when two or more services are furnished by the same physician to the same patient, in the same session, on the same day.

[h] See Medicare Payment Advisory Commission, Report to Congress: Aligning Incentives in Medicare (Washington, D.C.: June 2010).

[i] See Medicare Payment Advisory Commission, Report to the Congress: Medicare and the Healthcare Delivery System (Washington, D.C.: June 2011).

[j] See GAO, Medicare Part B Imaging Services: Rapid Spending Growth and Shift to Physician Offices Indicate Need for CMS to Consider Additional Management Practices, GAO-08-452 (Washington, D.C.: June 13, 2008).

[k] Donald H. Romano, "Self-Referral of Imaging and Increased Utilization: Some Practical Perspectives on Tackling the Dilemma," Journal of the American College of Radiology (2009): 773-779.

[l] The stated goal of the recovery audit program is to identify improper payments for services provided to Medicare beneficiaries. Improper payments may be overpayments or underpayments. Overpayments can occur when health care providers submit claims that do not meet Medicare's coding or medical necessity policies.

[m] Medicare Program; Changes to Disclosure of Physician Ownership in Hospitals and Physician Self-Referral Rules, 73 Fed. Reg. 48434, 48713 (Aug. 19, 2008).

[n] Medicare Program; Changes to Disclosure of Physician Ownership in Hospitals and Physician Self-Referral Rules, 73 Fed. Reg. 48434, 48719 (Aug. 18, 2008).

[o] Medicare Program; Proposed Revisions to Payment Policies Under the Physician Fee Schedule, and Other Part B Payment Policies for CY 2008, 72 Fed. Reg. 38122, 38181 (July 12, 2007).

[p] See Medicare Payment Advisory Commission, Report to Congress: Aligning Incentives in Medicare (Washington, D.C.: June 2010).

[q] Md. Code Ann., Health Occ. § 1-301(k)(2).

APPENDIX III: SELF-REFERRAL OF MRI AND CT SERVICES, BY PROVIDER SPECIALTY, IN 2004 AND 2010

The proportion of MRI services and CT services that were self-referred increased from 2004 through 2010 for all provider specialties we examined for our study. We examined all provider specialties that performed a minimum proportion of either self-referred MRI or CT services in 2004 and 2010.[1] While this increase across provider specialties is consistent with the overall trend of increased self-referral, the increases varied among provider specialties. For MRI services, increases in the self-referral rate for provider specialties ranged from about 4 percentage points (Internal Medicine) to about 19 percentage points for Hematology/Oncology. Similarly, for CT services, increases in the self-referral rates for provider specialties ranged from about 2 percentage points (Internal Medicine) to over 38 percentage points (Radiation Oncology). (see table 5).

Table 5. Self-referral Rates of MRI and CT Services for Select Provider Specialties

Specialty[a]	Percentage of MRI services self-referred in 2004	Percentage of MRI services self-referred in 2010	Change in MRI Self-referral rate from 2004 to 2010 (percentage points)	Percentage of CT services self-referred in 2004	Percentage of CT services self-referred in 2010	Change in CT self-referral rate from 2004 to 2010 (percentage points)
Cardiology	n/a	n/a	n/a	33.5 %	55.4%	21.9
Family Practice	10.8	15.7	4.8	25.0	27.6	2.6
Gastroenterology	n/a	n/a	n/a	18.5	24.0	5.5
General Surgery	n/a	n/a	n/a	21.5	24.8	3.3
Hematology/Oncology	15.3	34.3	19.0	39.8	48.7	9.0
Internal Medicine	12.1	16.1	4.0	27.2	29.0	1.8
Medical Oncology	n/a	n/a	n/a	39.7	51.7	12.0
Neurology	19.7	28.9	9.1	n/a	n/a	n/a
Neurosurgery	20.5	26.1	5.6	n/a	n/a	n/a
Physical Medicine	22.7	29.4	6.7	n/a	n/a	n/a
Orthopedic Surgery	27.1	38.4	11.4	n/a	n/a	n/a
Otolaryngology	n/a	n/a	n/a	21.3	32.4	11.1
Pulmonary Disease	n/a	n/a	n/a	27.8	29.7	1.9
Radiation Oncology	n/a	n/a	n/a	37.7	76.1	38.4
Rheumatology	29.4	38.6	9.2	n/a	n/a	n/a
Urology	n/a	n/a	n/a	27.8	51.2	23.4

Source: GAO analysis of Medicare data.

Notes: "n/a" indicates that the provider specialty referred less than1.5 percent of all self-referred services, for MRI or CT services, in either 2004 or 2010. If a provider specialty did not refer at least 1.5 percent of all self-referred services for both 2004 and 2010 for either MRI or CT services, it is not included in the table.

[a]Provider specialties are included in Medicare claims data and are self-reported.

End Notes

[1] Medicare is the federally financed health insurance program for persons aged 65 and over, certain individuals with disabilities, and individuals with end-stage renal disease. Medicare Part A covers hospital and other inpatient

stays. Medicare Part B is optional insurance, and covers physician, outpatient hospital, home health care, and certain other services. Medicare Parts A and B are known as original Medicare or Medicare fee-forservice (FFS).

[2] See The Boards of Trustees, 2012 Annual Report of the Boards of Trustees of the Federal Hospital Insurance and Federal Supplementary Medical Insurance Trust Funds (Washington, D.C.: April 2012). The projected Medicare Part B growth rate assumes that scheduled statutory cuts in physician payment rates will be overridden by Congress as they have been every year since 2003.

[3] See Bureau of Economic Analysis, "Gross Domestic Product (GDP) Percent change from preceding period," National Economic Accounts (Washington, D.C.: May 31, 2012), accessed June 27, 2012, http://www.bea.gov/national/xls/gdpchg.xls.

[4] See Congressional Budget Office, The Budget and Economic Outlook: Fiscal Years 2012 through 2022 (Washington, D.C.: January 2012).

[5] Other advanced imaging services include nuclear medicine services. For the purposes of this report, "advanced imaging services" refers to only MRI and CT services.

[6] For example, see Laurence C. Baker, "Acquisition of MRI Equipment by Doctors Drives Up Imaging Use and Spending," Health Affairs, vol. 29, no. 12 (2010); Medicare Payment Advisory Commission, Report to the Congress, Improving Incentives in the Medicare Program (Washington, D.C.: June 2009); and Senator Grassley Press Release, Grassley Works to Protect Medicare Dollars, Empower Patients with Information (July 25, 2008), accessed May 31, 2012. http://www.finance.senate.gov/newsroom/ ranking/release/?id= bb006ccf-dedc-40fd-9b14- 6074cb2687f3.

[7] Compliance with the physician self-referral law, commonly known as the Stark law, is outside the scope of this report. The Stark law prohibits physicians from making referrals for certain designated health services paid for by Medicare, to entities with which the physicians or immediate family members have a financial relationship, unless the arrangement complies with a specified exception, such as in-office ancillary services. 42 U.S.C. § 1395nn(b)(2).The requirements of the in-office ancillary services exception are found at 42 C. F. R. § 411.355(b) (2011).The Patient Protection and Affordable Care Act (PPACA) amended the Stark law to establish an additional requirement with respect to the in-office ancillary services exception for certain types of advanced imaging services. That is, self-referring physicians must inform patients in writing at the time of referral for these services that the patient may obtain the service from a person other than the referring physician or someone in the physician's group practice and provide the patient with a list of suppliers who furnish the service in the area in which the patient resides. Pub. L. No. 111-148, § 6003, 124 Stat. 119, 697 (codified at 42 U.S.C. § 1395nn(b)(2)).

[8] Pub. L. No. 109-171, § 5102(b), 120 Stat. 4, 39-40 (2006).

[9] See GAO, Medicare Part B Imaging Services: Rapid Spending Growth and Shift to Physician Offices Indicate Need for CMS to Consider Additional Management Practices, GAO-08-452 (Washington, D.C.: June 13, 2008).

[10] See Medicare Payment Advisory Commission, Report to the Congress: Medicare and the Healthcare Delivery System (Washington, D.C.: June 2011).

[11] In addition to this report on advanced imaging, we also have ongoing work related to the self-referral of anatomic pathology services, intensity-modulated radiation therapy services, and physical therapy services.

[12] For the purposes of our report, we limited MRI or CT services (1) to those that were designated health services—services which, in the absence of an exception, a physician may not make a referral to furnish to an entity with which he has a financial relationship without implicating the Stark law—and (2) to those where the service includes the performance of the imaging service—which can be billed with or separately from the interpretation of a MRI or CT imaging service.

[13] An indicator or "flag" could be, for example, a modifier that a provider lists on a claim to indicate that a service is self-referred. Providers currently use modifiers to provide additional information about a service to CMS. For example, if a provider is only billing for the technical component of an imaging service, the provider would use a modifier to alert CMS that the claim does not cover the professional component of the service.

[14] Providers could have a financial relationship with the same entity if, for example, they are part of the same group practice.

[15] IDTFs are diagnostic testing facilities that are independent of a physician's office or hospital and that comply with a number of requirements including those related to the use of qualified supervising physicians, qualified nonphysician personnel, performance of only specifically ordered tests, and compliance with all applicable state laws. See 42 C.F.R. § 410.33 (2011). Radiologists and providers in IDTFs predominantly perform

advanced imaging services and have limited ability to refer beneficiaries for advanced imaging services. These providers are unlikely to self-refer MRI or CT services.

[16] Providers can also provide advanced imaging services in settings other than physician offices or IDTFs, such as hospitals.

[17] We defined urban areas as metropolitan statistical areas, a geographic entity defined by the Office of Management and Budget as a core urban area of 50,000 or more population; all other settings are considered rural.

[18] Providers with a radiology or IDTF specialty were removed because they have limited ability to refer beneficiaries for advanced imaging services, and thus are not likely to self-refer MRI or CT services. We excluded emergency medicine providers from our analysis because they did not practice in provider offices. After we made our exclusions, there were 419,884 providers that referred at least one MRI service and 477,547 providers that referred at least one CT service in 2010.

[19] In 2010, 35,950 providers self-referred an MRI service and 39,913 providers self-referred a CT service. In comparison, there were 383,934 non-self-referring MRI providers and 437,634 non-self-referring CT providers.

[20] We defined physician specialty using the specialty codes included in the Medicare claims. These specialty codes include physician specialties, such as cardiology and hematology/oncology, and nonphysician provider types, such as nurse practitioners and physician assistants.

[21] The other four imaging modalities are nuclear medicine, ultrasound, X-ray and other standard imaging, and procedures that use imaging.

[22] Medicare Payment Advisory Commission, Report to Congress: Aligning Incentives in Medicare (Washington, D.C.: June 2010).

[23] As noted in the Scope and Methodology section, the universe of services for this finding refers to advanced imaging services performed in a provider's office or in an IDTF. We focused on these settings because our previous work showed rapid growth among such services and because the financial incentive for providers to self-refer is most direct when the service is performed in a physician office.

[24] Under a provision in the DRA, Medicare fees for certain imaging services covered by the Medicare physician fee schedule cannot exceed what Medicare pays under the hospital outpatient prospective payment system, effectively mandating reduction in fees for certain services. Pub. L. No. 109-171, § 5102(b), 120 Stat. 4, 39-40 (2006). See GAO, Medicare: Trends in Fees, Utilization, and Expenditures for Imaging Services before and after Implementation of the Deficit Reduction Act of 2005, GAO-08-1102R (Washington, D.C.: September 26, 2008).

[25] We included specialties that referred at least 1.5 percent of self-referred MRI or CT services in 2004 and 2010. Sixteen provider specialties met these criteria for MRI services, CT services, or both types of services. These specialties were Cardiology, Family Practice, Gastroenterology, General Surgery, Hematology/Oncology, Internal Medicine, Medical Oncology, Neurology, Neurosurgery, Physical Medicine, Pulmonary Disease, Orthopedic Surgery, Otolaryngology, Radiation Oncology, Rheumatology, and Urology.

[26] As discussed earlier, the scope of services included in this analysis is broader than our analysis of self-referred services. Specifically, this analysis includes settings other than a physician office or IDTF, such as a hospital. We did this to fully capture the advanced imaging referral patterns of self-referring and non-self-referring providers to ensure that the comparison between the groups was comparable.

[27] CMS has a long-standing policy called a multiple procedure payment reduction that is meant to avoid duplicate payments for expenses that are incurred only once when two or more surgical services are furnished together by the same physician during the same operating session. CMS expanded the multiple procedure payment reduction to include certain imaging services in 2006. Medicare Program: Revisions to Payment Policies Under the Physician Fee Schedule for Calendar Year 2006, 70 Fed. Reg. 70116 (Nov. 21, 2005). In our 2009 report, we recommended that CMS expand its efforts to ensure that fees for services paid under the physician fee schedule reflect efficiencies that occur when services are performed by the same physician to the same beneficiary on the same day. See GAO, Medicare Physician Payments: Fees Could Better Reflect Efficiencies Achieved When Services Are Provided Together, GAO-09-647 (Washington, D.C.: July 31, 2009). In 2012, CMS expanded its multiple procedure payment reduction policy by applying a reduction to the PC of imaging services that are provided during the same session, to the same patient, on the same day; the agency had previously applied the multiple procedure payment reduction to only the TC of imaging services that met the same criteria.

[28] We grouped providers of each specialty with at least 1,000 self-referring providers into five provider-size categories: (1) fewer than 50 unique Medicare FFS patients; (2) 51-100 unique Medicare FFS patients; (3)

101-250 unique Medicare FFS patients; (4) 251-500 unique Medicare FFS patients; and (5) more than 500 unique Medicare FFS patients. The seven specialties that had at least 1,000 self-referring providers were Family Practice, Hematology/Oncology, Internal Medicine, Neurology, Nurse Practitioners, Orthopedic Surgeons, and Physician Assistants.

[29] The nine specialties where self-referring providers referred more beneficiaries for CT services than non-self-referring providers across the majority of provider size categories were: Cardiology, Gastroenterology, General Surgery, Hematology/Oncology, Nurse Practitioners, Orthopedic Surgery, Otolaryngology, Urology, and Pulmonary Disease specialists. The four specialties where non-self-referring providers referred more beneficiaries for CT services, on average, than self-referring providers across the majority of provider size categories were Family Practice, Internal Medicine, Neurology, and Physician Assistants.

[30] We considered a provider to have remained in the same practice if the entity to which they most commonly referred MRI or CT services remained the same from 2007 through 2010.

[31] We limited our analysis to expenditures directly related to imaging services. There may be additional costs associated with the increased use of advanced imaging services by self-referring providers, if these imaging services reveal abnormalities that have no clinical relevance or result in unnecessary surgeries. In contrast, increased use of advanced imaging may partially offset some of these direct imaging costs if increased use led to the early detection of disease and resulted in less-invasive and less-costly treatments.

End Notes for Appendix I

[1] Services can have technical components (TC) and professional components (PC). The TC of a service is intended to cover the performance of a test, including the cost of equipment, supplies, and nonphysician staff. In addition, services have a PC, which for advanced imaging services is intended to cover the physician's time in interpreting an image and writing a report on the findings. The TC and PC of a service can be billed together on the same claim—called a global claim—or separately.

[2] The BETOS categorization system was developed by CMS primarily for analyzing the growth in Medicare expenditures by broad categories. Each billing code is assigned to only one BETOS category.

[3] Compliance with the physician self-referral law, commonly known as the Stark law, is outside the scope of this report. The Stark law prohibits physicians from making referrals for certain designated health services paid for by Medicare, to entities with which the physicians or immediate family members have a financial relationship, unless the arrangement complies with a specified exception, such as in-office ancillary services. 42 U.S.C. § 1395nn(b)(2).

[4] Some providers may be associated with TINs with which they do not have a direct or indirect financial relationship and thus would not have the same incentives as other self-referring providers. We anticipate that relatively few providers in our self-referring group meet this description but to the extent that they do, it may have limited the differences we found in utilization and expenditure rates between self-referring and non-self-referring providers.

[5] The final rule implementing the Health Insurance Portability and Accountability Act established the standard for a unique health identifier for health care providers for use in the health care system and announced the adoption of the NPI as that standard. HIPAA Administrative Simplification: Standard Unique Health Identifier for Health Care Providers, 69 Fed. Reg. 2424 (Jan. 23, 2004) (adding a new subpart D to 45 C.F.R. part 162). Performing physicians were required to include their NPI on any claim submitted to Medicare as of May 23, 2008. Prior to implementation of the NPI, Medicare required providers to submit another type of unique provider identifier called the unique physician identification number. Our methodology for identifying self-referred services was similar to the methodology used by MedPAC for its study of the effect of physician self-referral on use of imaging services within an episode. See Medicare Payment Advisory Commission: Report to the Congress: Improving Incentives in the Medicare Program (Washington, DC, June 2009).

[6] Providers in our analysis that could self-refer include primarily physicians, but also could include other providers, such as nurse practitioners and physician assistants.

[7] We considered a location with a rural-urban commuting area code of 1.0, 1.1, 2.0, 2.1, or 3.0 to be a metropolitan statistical area.

[8] We used 4 years of experience (2007 through 2010) to categorize providers even though we compared referrals in 2008 to 2010 because we wanted to ensure that providers that began self-referring in 2009 did not self-refer for at least the 2 prior years.

End Note for Appendix III

[1] Specifically, for MRI and CT services, we examined provider specialties that referred at least 1.5 percent of the MRI or CT services that were self-referred in both 2004 and 2010. Specialties we examined referred about 86 percent of self-referred MRI services in 2004 and about 81 percent of self-referred MRI services in 2010. These specialties referred about 82 percent of self-referred CT services in 2004 and about 88 percent of self-referred CT services in 2010.

INDEX

D

E

F

G

H

I

K

L

M

N

O

P

Q

R

S

T

U

V

W